The Scoliosis Handbook

A CONSULTATION WITH A SPECIALIST

Michael Neuwirth, M.D.

with Kevin Osborn

HENRY HOLT AND COMPANY

NEW YORK

Henry Holt and Company, Inc.
Publishers since 1866
115 West 18th Street
New York, New York 10011

Henry Holt® is a registered
trademark of Henry Holt and Company, Inc.

Published in Canada by Fitzhenry & Whiteside Ltd.,
195 Allstate Parkway, Markham, Ontario L3R 4T8.

Library of Congress Cataloging-in-Publication Data
Neuwirth, Michael.
The scoliosis handbook: a consultation with a specialist / by
Michael Neuwirth, with Kevin Osborn.—1st ed.
p.   cm.
Includes bibliographical references and index.
ISBN 0-8050-3793-4
1. Scoliosis—Popular works.   I. Osborn, Kevin, 1959—
II. Title.
RD771.S3N48   1996
617.3'75—dc20   95-32801
CIP

Henry Holt books are available for special promotions and premiums.
For details contact: Director, Special Markets.

First Edition—1996

Book design by Claire Naylon Vaccaro

Printed in the United States of America
All first editions are printed on acid-free paper. ∞

1   3   5   7   9   10   8   6   4   2

To Ronald DeWald, my teacher and mentor,
and to my wife, Linda, and my son, Evan,
for their constant support and encouragement.

—M.N.

To Susie, Megan, Ian, and Molly,
for their understanding, faith, and patience.

—K.O.

Contents

List of Illustrations

Acknowledgments

We would like to thank a number of people, without whose contributions this book would not have come to life: Raquel Jaramillo, who first saw a need for this book and got the ball rolling; Richard Parks, who brought us together on this project; Teresa Joyce, who deftly coordinated our schedules and kept us together; Jo Ann Haun at Henry Holt, who supported our work and nurtured it along; Elizabeth McGuinness of the Long Island Scoliosis Society, Joe O'Brien, president of the National Scoliosis Foundation, Keith H. Bridwell, M.D., of Barnes Hospital in St. Louis, and Andrew Meyers of Advanced Orthopedic Technologies, Inc., for sharing their time and expertise; and above all, the people who so generously shared their experiences and wisdom with us.

Introduction

Seventeen years ago when I started my practice, I was constantly asked by patients for literature that they might read on scoliosis, its prognosis, its natural history, and its treatment alternatives. It became quickly apparent to me that no good resource existed for patients to use to answer these questions. The available literature was either written for a professional audience and too technical, or written for young children and too basic, or simply out of date. I strongly believe that the more knowledgeable and better educated my patients are about their condition, the more effectively they can be treated.

I had often thought about writing a book on scoliosis, but never seemed to have the opportunity. With the encouragement and support of my patients, my family, and my editor, this book became a reality and I am very happy with the result. It sounds like me sitting in my office talking with a patient, and that is exactly what we were striving for. I hope that you find the information in this book useful, and if scoliosis treatment is needed, reassuring.

MICHAEL NEUWIRTH, M.D.
Chief of Spine Services
The Hospital for Joint Diseases
New York City

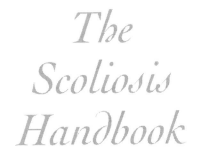

The
Scoliosis
Handbook

CHAPTER ONE

What Is Scoliosis?

"WE WENT ON A RETREAT THIS YEAR AND EACH OF us had to talk about life experiences," begins Susannah, a charming, intelligent, and lovely girl of 17. "And I was asked, 'What was the worst experience of your life? And what was the best experience of your life?' and I said, 'Well, it was the same thing.' Having this operation really was the worst and the best. The worst because I had to go through more than what I should have had to go through at that age in terms of being afraid and thinking about it. But it was the best in that I think largely who I am today is first of all because of the fact that this long-term crisis made me realize how special my family and my friends are to me and how they all pulled for me and were so loyal and gave me so much love. Number two, it made me who I am because I had to think about these scary things and be brave and be grown up at a time when it would have been easier to just be a teenager. It made me really appreciate that being healthy is the most you can ask for. So I'm glad it happened. It's definitely something I'm proud of."

If you have just been diagnosed with scoliosis, or if you have recently learned that your child has scoliosis, chances are you don't share Susannah's perspective. When first diagnosed with any disease, many patients can only see the worst. You may not know what to think. Betty, now in her mid-fifties, remembers her reaction when, at age 12, she learned she had scoliosis: "The doctors tried to explain, but we were at a loss because we had never heard of anybody with it. We didn't know what it was. We just knew it was a very deforming, crippling disease." Like Betty and most of the other patients whom I treat for scoliosis, you probably have many questions: What is scoliosis? How did I get it? Will I be permanently disfigured? Can anything make it go away? What can be done about it? Will it create other health problems for me? How will it affect my future?

What Is Scoliosis?

Scoliosis, a term (meaning "crookedness" in Greek) first used by the ancient Greek physician Galen more than 18 centuries ago, is most simply defined as a lateral (side-to-side rather than front-to-back) curvature of the spine. When looked at from the front or from behind, the spine should be perfectly straight. But the scoliotic spine curves either to one side or first to one side and then to the other.

As you read about scoliosis, you should keep in mind that although the sideways curvature that characterizes scoliosis marks a deviation from the normal spine, the spine is *not* normally straight from all vantage points. When viewed from the side, the spine normally has several curves. The *lumbar spine*, the portion of the spine located in the lower back, should have some degree of *lordosis*: When viewed from the side, the lumbar spine curves forward, creating an indentation on the surface of the lower back. By contrast, the *thoracic spine*, the region of the spine situated in the middle and upper back, normally demonstrates a slight *kyphosis*: It rounds outward, toward the surface of the back. Normal lumbar lordosis and thoracic kyphosis (also called *sagittal curves*) help maintain balance and keep us upright. Indeed, either a loss or an exaggerated degree of lordosis and kyphosis can significantly impede an individual's balance. So some degree of spinal curvature is normal and has a function. In a perfect spine, however, there should be no *lateral* deviation from the straight line.

Not everyone whose spine curves from side to side is diagnosed with scoliosis. Orthopedists (doctors specializing in the correction and prevention of skeletal deformities) determine the magnitude of a scoliotic curve by measuring what's known as the Cobb angle. To measure the Cobb angle, lines are drawn on a spinal X-ray parallel to the highest and lowest vertebrae involved in a scoliotic curve. In a straight spine, both of these lines would be horizontal. Next, a line is drawn perpendicular to each of those lines. The angle of intersection of those two perpendiculars equals the magnitude of the curve. In a straight spine, these perpendiculars would be parallel vertical lines and the Cobb angle would be 0 degrees. Spinal curves of less than 10 degrees, which generally entail little risk of growing larger, are not considered scoliosis by orthopedists. This number is somewhat arbitrary, a line in the sand that helps determine the magnitude of curve that warrants treatment or, at the very least, further observation. Some people not diagnosed with scoliosis may have minor spinal curves, but medical professionals do not regard such curves as causes for concern.

As the spine curves, deviating to the side, it also tends to rotate—the vertebrae rotate on their axis. This rotation of the vertebrae, rather than the curve itself, creates the most noticeable physical characteristic of pronounced scoliosis: the rib hump that projects from the plane of the back. Other physical signs often escape notice. One shoulder blade may be higher than the other. The waistline may be asymmetrical, causing pants or skirts to hang unevenly. Although these signs of scoliosis can easily be overlooked, ignored, minimized, or rationalized, a significant rib hump seldom goes undetected. Clinically defined, then, scoliosis means *the presence of a lateral deviation of 10 degrees or more in the spine, often associated with rotation of the vertebrae.*

Should spinal curvature and rib rotation—the defining characteristics of scoliosis—warrant concern? Not always. Most people with scoliosis live lives as full, active, and unrestricted as those with straight spines. But for about 10 percent of those who have the condition, scoliosis leads to physical problems, chronic pain, and/or medical complications that require surgical or nonsurgical intervention. Whether you or your child falls into the former or the latter group depends on the size of the curve, its location, and the rate of its progression—how fast it is growing.

Types of Scoliosis

Orthopedists attempt to classify different types of scoliosis according to the cause of the deformity, but by far the most common type of scoliosis, accounting for 80 to 85 percent of all cases, is *idiopathic scoliosis; idiopathic* means that we don't know what causes it. Idiopathic scoliosis is a diagnosis of exclusion: When doctors have ruled out all specific causes of a case of scoliosis, they categorize that scoliosis as idiopathic. Except for the curvature in the spine, the child or adult is perfectly normal. At birth, the child's spine was straight. And though the doctor identifies nothing else as abnormal, the spine has grown in a crooked way for reasons not yet understood.

Orthopedists refer to four different types of idiopathic scoliosis, classified according to the age of the patient when the curvature first appeared:

1. *Infantile idiopathic scoliosis* first appears before the child's third birthday. Very rare in the United States today, infantile idiopathic scoliosis is a disease that is genetically different from the other types of idiopathic scoliosis. Yet because the cause remains unknown, it can only be called idiopathic.

2. *Juvenile idiopathic scoliosis* develops between the ages of three and ten. Although arbitrarily distinguished from adolescent idiopathic scoliosis (see below), juvenile idiopathic scoliosis is probably the same disease under a different name. Both result in very similar curve patterns. Even so, the distinction is significant. Since children diagnosed with idiopathic scoliosis before age 10 have so many more years of growth remaining than those diagnosed during adolescence, children with juvenile idiopathic scoliosis have a much greater risk of significant curve progression.

3. *Adolescent idiopathic scoliosis*, the most common type of scoliosis, typically appears between the ages of 10 and 13—at or near the onset of puberty. Like juvenile idiopathic scoliosis,

adolescent idiopathic scoliosis typically causes no significant pain during childhood.

4. *Adult idiopathic scoliosis*, most likely adolescent idiopathic scoliosis continued into adulthood, is marked by significant curve progression following the completion of physical maturity. Although adult idiopathic scoliosis may not be detected until adulthood, it may nonetheless have been present but undiagnosed during childhood.

In only 15 to 20 percent of scoliosis cases has a cause been identified. These types of scoliosis include congenital scoliosis, neuromuscular scoliosis, and degenerative scoliosis.

Congenital scoliosis, present at birth, results from birth defects that create abnormalities in the way the spine is segmented or from failures of certain portions of the spine to form. These spinal malformations result in asymmetric spinal growth, thereby producing scoliosis. Much more disparate in the way it presents than idiopathic scoliosis, congenital scoliosis is often associated with other problems, such as kidney dysfunctions, urinary-tract abnormalities, or congenital heart defects.

Neuromuscular scoliosis is caused by one or more neuromuscular diseases that result in inadequate functioning of the nerves and/or muscles around the spine. Prior to the mid-1950s, poliomyelitis (polio), a virus that causes inflammation in the spinal cord, accounted for most cases of neuromuscular scoliosis. Today, most neuromuscular scolioses develop as a result of cerebral palsy, a disability that results from damage to the brain's motor centers, or muscular dystrophy, a disease marked by progressive wasting of muscles throughout the body.

Degenerative scoliosis (see Chapter 8) forms during adult life in a previously straight spine as a result of a degeneration of the discs, arthritis in the facet joints (the joints that link vertebral segments of the spine), and/or loss of support in the spinal column. In older patients, differentiating between worsening idiopathic scoliosis and true degenerative scoliosis becomes difficult. A small idiopathic curve that develops degenerative changes as a result of aging can closely resemble a true degenerative scoliosis. However, the more angular curves that characterize degenerative scoliosis generally involve fewer vertebrae than the longer curves of idiopathic scoliosis. Also, degenerative curves tend to be smaller than those resulting from idiopathic scoliosis. Despite the smaller length and magnitude of degenerative curves, degenerative scoliosis is more commonly associated with pain and discomfort than idiopathic scoliosis.

No matter what type of scoliosis you or your child may have, the disease has altered the shape of the spine. As mentioned earlier, this curvature does not have a significant impact on most people with scoliosis. With a minor spinal curve, you can do everything that someone else with no curve can do. But if the curve grows progressively larger, it can create other, more troublesome problems.

How Scoliosis Affects the Anatomy of the Back

In order to understand scoliosis, you'll first need to know a little about the anatomy of the back. The human spinal column consists of 24 vertebrae, flexible bony elements that rise from the *sacrum* and *coccyx*. (See Figure 1.) The coccyx, more commonly known as the tailbone, and the sacrum together function as a

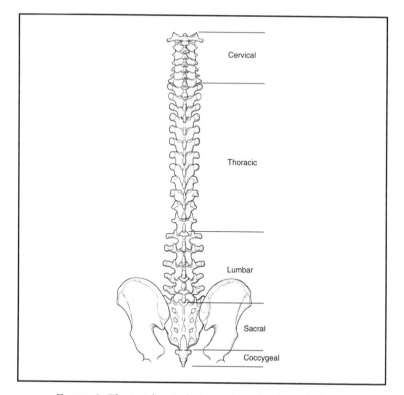

FIGURE 1. *The straight spinal column illustrating the cervical spine, the thoracic spine, the lumbar spine, the sacrum, and the pelvis.*

stable post upon which the rest of the vertebrae sit and actually consist of vertebrae themselves. But the five vertebrae of the sacrum and the four vertebrae of the coccyx have fused together to form two solid, inflexible bones.

Rising from the base of the sacrum and coccyx, the 24 other vertebrae remain separate and flexible. These 24 vertebrae are classified and numbered from top to bottom, according to three regions of the spinal column. Seven *cervical* vertebrae form the top of the spinal column, ranging from C1 attached to the cranium or skull to C7 at the base of the neck. Below these are the 12 thoracic vertebrae, which support the ribs, with T1 located just below the neck and T12 connected to the highest lumbar vertebra (L1). The lumbar spine consists of five vertebrae located in the lower back, with L1 at the top of the lower back and L5 attached to the sacrum.

Each vertebra is joined to the one below it and the one above it by a three-joint complex. A *disc*, which lies between two vertebrae at the front of the spine, consists of a fibrous cartilage ring that surrounds a soft, spongy core and serves as a shock absorber for the spine. Each vertebra also has two *facet joints*, located at the back of the spine. The superior facet joint unites a vertebra with the one above it, and the inferior facet joint joins it with the vertebra below. The disc and facet joints work together to provide both stability and mobility to the spine.

Together, the vertebrae and joints of the spinal column serve a number of important functions. They provide a point of attachment for various muscles, thereby allowing motion and flexibility to the back and torso. They support all the weight of the upper part of the body. And they provide protection to the spinal cord, the main pathway traveled by nerve impulses on their way to or from the brain. In order to fulfill all of these functions, the spinal column must remain strong, flexible, and durable.

Mild cases of scoliosis, as well as the mild early stages of more severe cases, have no effect on the functioning of the spine and back. Indeed, most people with scoliosis function perfectly normally. Mild scoliosis does not interfere with the spine's flexibility or stability or its ability to bear weight or to protect the spinal cord. So in its early stages and in minor cases, scoliosis has no further effects than to cause asymmetry or deformity in the shape of the spine.

As time goes on and scoliotic curves get larger, however, they can create additional problems that *do* impair functioning. More severe scoliosis can create postural imbalance, where the head is no longer centered over the pelvis. This imbalance can force back muscles to work harder to maintain an erect posture and to fight the effects of gravity. This extra effort may lead to increased muscle fatigue and pain.

In addition, the imbalance may lead to arthritic changes (inflammation and enlargement of the joints) in the back, which may also result in heightened pain and/or stiffness. Patients with severe scoliosis often develop *spondylosis*, arthritis of the spine. In general, the larger the curve, the more arthritic the patient will become. As curves get larger and more asymmetrical, the abnormal stresses they place on discs may cause this arthritis. Discs degenerate, narrow, and lose water content; collagen fibers in the disk break apart; facet joints become hypertrophic (enlarged); osteophytes (bone spurs) form on the facet joints; and cartilage, which normally glistens to allow for smooth motion, becomes pitted and thin. In the worst arthritic cases, with no joint left at all, the spine spontaneously fuses, making movement impossible. Although the incidence of spondylosis does not differ significantly among scoliotic and nonscoliotic patients, those with scoliosis tend to have more advanced degrees of spondylosis, more pain associated with arthritis, and less responsiveness to appropriate nonoperative treatments such as exercise, physical therapy, and pain medications. I have operated on patients as young as 15 years old who have had advanced arthritic changes in their thoracic spines owing to severe scoliosis, changes that brought on significant pain problems. Indeed, virtually all the adults with scoliosis whom I have treated surgically have had some arthritic changes in their spines.

If curves, especially those located in the thoracic region of the spine, get very large, scoliosis can also begin to affect the functioning of the lungs and even the heart. These secondary respiratory complications, known as restrictive lung disease, can make breathing difficult and thereby decrease the amount of oxygen sent from the lungs to the heart. Fortunately, such complications have become increasingly rare in patients with idiopathic scoliosis. Scoliotic curves must get very large, greater than 100 degrees, before a person will develop any significant cardiopulmonary problems. A lesser curve may still cause some changes in pulmonary function, but these changes do not become significantly troublesome unless the curve approaches or exceeds 100 degrees. And either because most curves today are caught early and treated appropriately or because scoliosis behaves differently today than it once did, the number of curves that progress to that size is now very small.

Scoliosis can also lead to neurological problems such as nerve-root compression. As they exit from the spinal canal, nerves need space in which to function freely. If pinched because of lack of space, this nerve-root compression may cause pain, numbness, weakness, or tingling that typically runs down into the legs. Impairment of nerve functioning, however, occurs rarely as a result of idiopathic scoliosis. More commonly it results from degenerative scoliosis, generally accompanied by disc collapse and/or arthritis, which often compromises space that normally should be available for the nerves.

Types of Curves

Now that you know the different types and causes of scoliosis and a little about the basic structure of the spine, let's look at the various types of spinal curves that can form. Scoliotic curves are defined by location, shape, and magnitude, or the size of the angle. Since curves always involve more than one vertebra, orthopedists pinpoint the location of the curve by referring to the end vertebrae and the apex of the curve. For example, a curve described as having endpoints at T4 and T10 with an apex at T7 extends from the fourth thoracic vertebra to the tenth and deviates farthest from the center line of the back at the seventh thoracic vertebra. A typical idiopathic thoracic curve will span six to eight vertebrae, and a typical lumbar curve will involve four vertebrae.

The four most common curve patterns caused by idiopathic scoliosis (see Figures 2 A–D) are:

1. *Thoracic curves.* As their name suggests, single thoracic curves occur in the thoracic spine. Ninety percent of thoracic curves have right convexity: Looked at from the back, the spine curves to the right before rounding back toward the midline of the back.

2. *Thoracolumbar curves.* These curves span both the thoracic and the lumbar spine, with the apex located at the junction between the thoracic and the lumbar spine. Eighty percent of thoracolumbar curves demonstrate right convexity.

3. *Lumbar curves.* Lumbar curves are situated entirely within the five vertebrae of the lumbar spine. Unlike thoracic and thoracolumbar curves, however, the majority (70 percent) of

FIGURE 2. *Line drawings that accompany the X-rays on the following two pages illustrate the asymmetry of the trunk. Each curve pattern causes a different type of asymmetrical appearance to the back. The heavy black lines illustrate the end points of the curve and the numbers indicating the Cobb angles are written over the apical vertebra.*

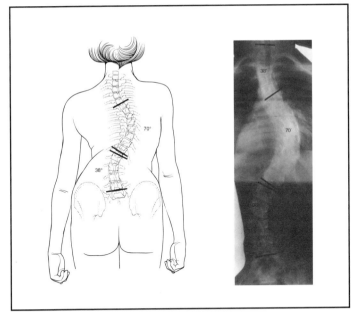

A. Right thoracic curve. It measures 70 degrees by the Cobb method.

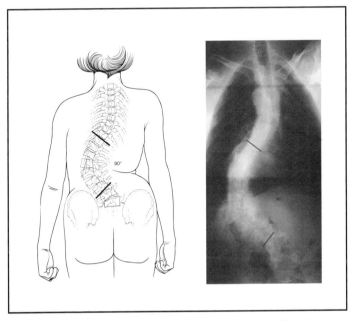

B. Thoracolumbar curve. It measures 90 degrees by the Cobb method.

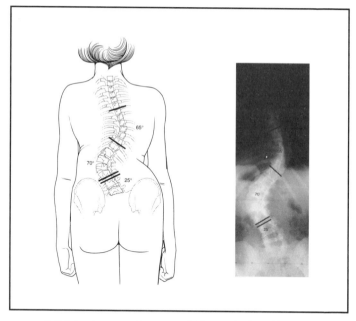

C. Left lumbar curve. It measures 70 degrees by the Cobb method.

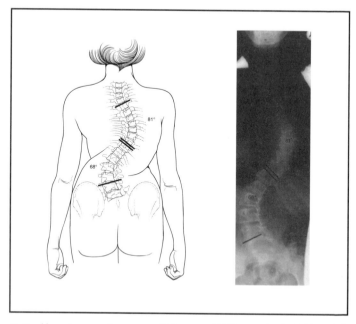

D. Double major curve. It measures 81 degrees and 68 degrees by the Cobb method.

lumbar curves exhibit left convexity, curving away from the spine toward the left.

4. *Double-major curves.* Double-major curves deviate from the straight spine in the shape of an **S** rather than a **C**. Two curves form, one with its apex to the right of the midline, the other with its apex to the left. Most typically, the right curve occurs in the thoracic spine and the left in the lumbar region.

These four types probably account for 95 percent of all scoliotic curves. Less common curves include double thoracic curves, two curves situated entirely within the thoracic spine; cervicothoracic curves, which deviate along both the cervical and high thoracic spine; and thoracic thoracolumbar curves, double curves with one apex in the thoracic spine and the other apex at the thoracolumbar junction. In my practice, whenever I am confronted with anything as rare as these curves, I generally suspect that an identifiable cause of the scoliosis exists. For instance, although cervicothoracic curves can be idiopathic, I always look carefully for an underlying cause when presented with a significant cervicothoracic curve because this type of curve is so uncommon as to raise suspicion. With the four most common curves I much more readily apply the idiopathic designation, although I also consider carefully the possibility of an underlying cause.

Who Gets Scoliosis?

Until the recent advent of screening programs for scoliosis in the schools, no one knew the prevalence of scoliosis in the general population of adolescents or adults. Many cases of adolescent idiopathic scoliosis went undetected, because it rarely causes any symptoms—any actual physical complaints—among adolescents. Even kids with curves measuring as high as 80 degrees often have no symptoms other than the deformity itself, or perhaps a little muscular backache. And this back pain may be entirely unrelated to the scoliosis, since back pain from a number of causes is prevalent in the general population. An adolescent with scoliosis may occasionally notice that he looks a little misshapen. The child or a parent may notice an unevenness in the hips, since scoliotic spine curves often result in noticeable asymmetry in the level of the hips. But in most cases, adolescent idiopathic scoliosis presents no symptoms whatsoever that demand attention. School screenings for scoliosis, now required in more than 30 states, not only have increased general awareness of scoliosis, but have also provided us much more information on the prevalence and distribution of scoliosis in adolescent populations.

What have we learned? Anyone can develop scoliosis. Yet since no one knows what causes idiopathic scoliosis, we also know little that anyone can do to reduce the risk of developing it. Indeed, the only known risk factor of real significance is something that we have no control over: Scoliosis tends to run in families. One study of the families of children with idiopathic scoliosis found that the incidence of scoliosis in the family members of these patients was 6 to 10 times higher than it was in the general population. This heightened risk of developing scoliosis is present not only in the children of parents with scoliosis but also in siblings, even if neither parent has scoliosis.

Overall, according to the Scoliosis Research Society of the American Academy of Orthopaedic Surgeons, about 10 percent of the adolescent population has some degree of scoliosis. Yet most of these have very small curves that require no treatment at all. Fewer than 10 percent of those diagnosed with scoliosis will ever require any treatment other than periodic examinations to watch for signs of curve progression. Only one out of two to three hundred 10-to-16-year-olds have curves greater than 20 degrees—i.e., curves requiring some medical attention, if only continued observation. Fewer than 1 percent of adolescents have curves exceeding 30 degrees. And less than one in one thousand children in this age group have curves that measure more than 40 degrees. Although I treat scoliosis patients every day, I very rarely see curves greater than 100 degrees these days.

Surprisingly, given that many people regard scoliosis as a disease that primarily afflicts females, the incidence of scoliosis is almost *equally* distributed among males and females. The general impression that girls get scoliosis far more than boys arises from the fact that statistically girls' spinal curves tend to *progress* (to increase in size over time) more frequently, more rapidly, and more significantly than boys' curves. A 12-year-old boy with a 10-degree thoracic curve has only about one-tenth the risk of progression as a girl of the same age who has a comparable curve. Among those whose curves grow large enough to require treatment, females outnumber males by about five to one. Exactly why curves progress more significantly in girls and women than in boys and men, we don't know.

The Progression of Scoliotic Curves

Just as we know little about what causes most types of scoliosis, we also know little about what causes some curves to progress rapidly and significantly and other curves to remain stable. But we do know that certain factors heighten the risk of curve *progression*, which is clinically defined as a documented 5-degree increase in the magnitude of the curve in two or more visits to the orthopedist. (These visits may be three months apart or three years apart, depending on the age of the patient and the size of the initial curve.) These risk factors include:

- *Gender.* As mentioned above, girls' scoliotic curves tend to progress more frequently and more severely than boys' curves. All other factors being equal, girls with scoliosis have a 10 times higher risk of curve progression than boys.

- *Age.* The younger the patient at the time of detection and diagnosis, the greater the risk of progression. According to data compiled for the Scoliosis Research Society, a child 10 to 12 years old who has a curve that measures between 20 and 29 degrees has a 60 percent risk of curve progression. For a child 13 to 15 years old with a comparable curve, the risk of progression drops down to 40 percent. And a child of 16 with a similar curve has only a 10 percent risk of progression.

  Actually, the decisive factor here lies not so much in the chronological age of the patient as in the child's skeletal maturity. Scoliosis tends to progress most rapidly during the preadolescent growth spurt, the years leading up to physical maturity. Rapid progression of scoliotic curves is associated with the rate of spinal growth during these years. This growth—and hence the risk of curve progression—usually peaks for girls between the ages of 10 and 14, after the development of breasts and pubic hair has begun, but prior to the onset of the first period. Among boys, spinal growth and risk of curve progression peak later, generally between the ages of 13 and 16, usually just prior to the development of facial hair.

- *Curve size.* The size of the curve when first diagnosed is also a significant indicator of the risk of progression. The larger the curve, the greater the risk. Returning to the example above, the 13-to-15-year-old with a 20-to-29-degree curve who has a 40 percent risk of progression would have only a 10 percent risk if the curve measured less than 20 degrees. When the magnitude of the curve is 30 to 59 degrees, the risk increases to 60 percent. And if that same child had a curve that exceeded 60 degrees, the risk of progression would skyrocket to 90 percent.
- *Curve pattern and location.* The type of curve also affects the risk of progression. Double curves have a significantly higher risk of progressing than single curves. Also, thoracic curves tend to progress more than lumbar curves. Thoracic curves of 50 to 80 degrees at skeletal maturity have the greatest risk of progression of any type of curve.

Our increasing knowledge of the risk factors associated with the progression of scoliotic curves has also led to the elimination of certain factors once thought to be linked to curve progression. We now know that a family history of scoliosis, which does significantly increase the risk of a family member developing scoliosis, apparently has no impact on whether that scoliosis will progress. Despite popular belief, the amount a person exercises, an individual's weight and muscle tone, and the amount of arthritis a person has also have no documented relation to curve progression.

Although curves progress most rapidly during the adolescent growth spurt, they do not necessarily stop progressing once a person has reached skeletal maturity. One study found that approximately two-thirds of the scoliosis patients followed over a 40-year period experienced curve progression after skeletal maturity. In general, curves that measure less than 30 degrees at skeletal maturity have no significant risk of progression. Indeed, many of these patients will not even require regular follow-up exams. Curves of 50 degrees or more have the greatest risk of progression during adulthood. Thoracic curves of this magnitude tend to progress an average of 1 to 3 degrees per year. But as curves become very large (75 to 80 degrees), the risk and rate of progression go down.

In weighing potential risk factors that might apply to *you*, you should remember that no "typical" progression exists. Each individual curve in each individual patient has its own natural history. Though statistics indicate what has happened to large groups of patients, they cannot predict what will happen to a specific individual. There is no way to predict absolutely from looking at an X-ray who will progress and who will not. The incidence and rate of curve progression varies greatly from person to person. While I might be able to tell you that on the basis of your age and gender as well as the size and type of your curve, *statistically* your curve has an 80 percent chance of progression, I cannot say whether you as an individual fall into the 80 percent whose curves do progress or the 20 percent whose curves do not.

What Might Cause Scoliosis?

My patients sometimes ask me what caused them to develop scoliosis. They want to know if anything they did might have caused the scoliosis — or if they might have done something differently that would have prevented the curve.

In cases involving nonidiopathic scolioses, I can readily provide answers. Congenital scoliosis begins at birth: Children are born with an abnormal spinal column that grows asymmetrically. Neuromuscular scolioses result from some abnormality in the neuromuscular system: abnormal control of muscles in the case of cerebral palsy, muscle paralysis due to an intrinsic muscle disorder in the case of muscular dystrophy. Degenerative scoliosis stems from deterioration of the discs that cushion the vertebrae, arthritis in the facet joints, and/or loss of support in the spinal column.

With idiopathic scolioses, however, the answers do not come as easily. Everything from poor posture to poor nutrition has been suggested as a possible cause. Today, most researchers exploring possible causes of scoliosis fall into one of two schools of thought.

The neurological, or neuromuscular, school considers scoliosis a secondary development resulting from an as-yet-undefined deficit or disease in the neuromuscular system. The underlying neurological defect or abnormality, according to these researchers, may involve motor control mechanisms or postural control mechanisms. This neurological dysfunction leads to abnormalities or anomalies in the muscles surrounding the spine. The abnormal action of these muscles then creates tension and exerts force that causes the spine to curve.

The second school of thought ascribes the origins of scoliosis to mechanical forces on the spine. Since the spine is a column, people in this school apply mechanical principles to explain how a column bends. The spinal column, like the columns in classical architecture, is exposed to a variety of forces that act on it. According to researchers exploring possible mechanical causes of scoliosis, some spinal columns are unable to maintain their shape in the face of forces such as gravity, the weight of the upper body, and movement.

Though I don't know what causes scoliosis, I do know some of the right questions to ask. Any explanation of the causes of idiopathic scoliosis needs to account for the following:

- *Why do more severe curves tend to afflict girls rather than boys?* Researchers have not yet pinpointed which of the many differences between boys and girls might contribute to the higher incidence and faster rate of progression of scoliotic curves in girls. It could be that hormonal differences exacerbate scoliosis or accelerate curve progression in girls. Or these differences might be related to the fact that girls go through their growth spurt and achieve physical maturity at an earlier age than boys.

- *Why do girls who get scoliosis tend to be taller and thinner than girls of the same age who don't have the condition?* Girls who develop adolescent idiopathic scoliosis tend to grow faster sooner than girls of the same age who maintain straight spines. The answer may lie in certain growth hormones that some researchers have associated with scoliosis, but what role these hormones might play in the development of scoliosis remains uncertain.

- *Why are right thoracic curves so much more common than any of the other curves?* No one knows why the thoracic spine is apparently more vulnerable to scoliotic developments than the lumbar or cervical spines, or why the vast majority of thoracic curves bend to the right. Complete answers to these questions would bring us much closer to understanding the origins of scoliosis itself.

- *Why does the statistical risk of developing scoliosis increase so dramatically among family members of those who have scoliosis?* The increased risk for family members of scoliosis patients would seem to suggest a genetic component to the etiology (development) of the disease. Since scoliosis does not follow a simple pattern of inheritance, a single gene that causes the disease seems an unlikely possibility. A more probable explanation involves the interaction of a number of different genes or a combination of genetic and environmental factors. If such genes or biochemical sequences do exist, however, neither they nor any possible environmental factors that might combine to cause the development of idiopathic scoliosis have yet been identified.

Researchers *have* uncovered factors linked to scoliosis: differences in disc contents (e.g., higher-than-normal collagen levels); hyperactive muscles adjacent to a scoliotic curve; higher-than-normal calcium concentrations in muscles around the vertebrae. Yet all of these factors raise chicken-and-egg problems: Which came first? No evidence has yet proved that abnormalities of muscle, disc, bone, and collagen common among scoliosis patients are not a result of the scoliosis itself, rather than a cause. Unfortunately, despite the best efforts of countless scoliosis researchers, the cause or causes of idiopathic scoliosis remain unknown.

CHAPTER TWO

The Importance
of Early Detection
and Treatment

"WHEN I WAS ABOUT THIRTEEN," REMEMBERS RACHEL, today a 31-year-old art director for a major publisher, "I noticed as I was looking in the mirror one day that one hip seemed slightly higher than the other. My mother immediately took me to the doctor and the doctor sent me to an orthopedist. The orthopedist told me that it looked like I had a slight case of scoliosis, which we would have to watch. If it became worse, I'd probably have to wear a brace. Well, it was watched and within about a year, they decided I should wear a Milwaukee brace.

"It was something I was rather embarrassed about and I don't understand that now. In fact, even with my closest friends, it's not something I've ever discussed. I'm really usually pretty open about things, but I felt in a sense like it was my own little private deformity, which I didn't want to share with any-body."

If you have recently learned that your child has scoliosis and the child is still in the early teen or preteen years, your child is really one of the lucky ones. Of course, like Rachel, your child may not feel at all lucky. She may feel self-conscious, deformed, embarrassed, even ashamed. But if your child has scoliosis, it won't go away by itself. Not knowing about it will neither halt nor correct the progression of spinal curves. In fact, scoliosis that goes undiagnosed is more likely to get worse than scoliosis monitored and treated appropriately by an orthopedist.

In general, the earlier idiopathic scoliosis is identified, the more time there is to treat the curve nonsurgically. Small curves found in young people are much more amenable to simple forms of treatment than curves found later that are larger. Detecting a curve before a child's skeletal structure has matured leaves all treatment options open. Once the child's bones have matured, bracing the back in an attempt to stabilize the curve and halt progression is no longer a viable option. Detecting scoliosis early may thus prevent the onset of more significant secondary symptoms or even the need for surgery down the line.

Since it seldom causes pain during childhood, idiopathic sco-liosis is usually noticed inadvertently. A doctor or nurse may no-tice curvature in the course of a regular physical, a school physical, or a physical prior to a child's going to camp. X-rays taken as precautions following a car accident or other physical trauma may reveal scoliosis. Occasionally, a parent (or children themselves) may notice when the child wears a bathing suit that the waistline seems atilt or one shoulder seems higher than the other—features that clothing can often conceal. A lot of parents, though, never see their preteen or teenage children undressed, in their underwear, or even in a bathing suit. This understandable concession to the growing child's modesty and need for privacy makes it much more difficult for parents to notice scoliotic curves in their adolescent children.

Fortunately, more than 30 states now recommend or require screening for scoliosis to take place through the school system. The programs now in place train nurses or gym teachers to do a brief scoliosis screening of all children, usually in the sixth or seventh grade. The nurses or teachers take a course that instructs them on how to use a *scoliometer*, a simple screening tool that somewhat resembles a carpenter's level, to detect spinal rotation. Studies have shown that nurses and even those not in the health professions can learn to do this screening test very well. One study found that public-health nurses trained to screen children for scoliosis were able to detect all curves greater than 20 degrees. Although school screening will not cut the incidence of scoliosis, it may reduce the number of large curves through early detection and treatment.

School screening does have several drawbacks, though. The biggest disadvantage is the cost involved. Many school systems simply don't have the money to pay for screening programs. In addition, children who test positive in a scoliosis screening must then consult an orthopedic specialist, at further cost to their families. Another problem lies in the lack of nationwide guidelines for screening. Some states have instituted parameters so broad—for example, California recommends referral for *any* amount of asymmetry detected in the thoracic or lumbar spine—that the number of false positive results and incidence of overreferral skyrockets. Children and their parents end up wasting time and money on an unnecessary consultation with an orthopedist who will tell them either that the child does not have scoliosis or that the degree of scoliosis does not warrant either treatment or follow-up observation.

Despite these shortcomings, I remain an advocate of school screening for all preadolescents and adolescents. Since idiopathic scoliosis is typically asymptomatic, screening can catch many cases of scoliosis *before* they progress to the point of needing surgery. True, most scoliotic curves don't require treatment. A small curve that progresses little during adolescence will likely remain a small curve during adult life, never creating a problem. Yet some curves do progress, and as they do, the incidence of problems rises. If curves go undetected (a possibility that school screening aims to prevent), there is no chance of halting the progression of scoliosis, progression that may increase the risk of complications associated with larger curves. Screening and early treatment for scoliosis do have a value worth the costs entailed: Screening picks up curves while they are still small, making possible measures that attempt to prevent them from becoming large curves requiring surgery. A Swedish study on the impact of that country's widespread school screening found that while the number of kids treated with braces increased, the severity of curves and hence the number of surgeries decreased significantly. Wouldn't you prefer to know about your child's scoliosis early enough to take measures that might help avoid the need for surgery?

Overall, I believe school screening has proved itself to be an efficient and effective tool. The question then becomes *when* to conduct such screening. The types of scoliosis that present before adolescence (congenital scoliosis or juvenile idiopathic scoliosis) are much less common and less difficult to detect through other means. Consequently, if conducted too early, the test misses too many kids who may later develop idiopathic scoliosis. Adolescent idiopathic scoliosis, the most common type of scoliosis, by definition doesn't occur until the preteen years (10, 11, 12 years old). If done too late, the screening will pick up all the kids who have scoliosis, but the opportunity to treat any of these children nonsurgically will have been lost. Although the Scoliosis Research Society recommends that all children be screened annually from age 10 to 14, this seems a little overcautious. Along with the American Academy of Orthopaedic Surgeons, I would advise screening for girls at ages 11 and 13 and for boys at age 13 or 14.

The rationale behind scoliosis screening is that by catching curves early, measures can be taken to halt progression before it causes complications or warrants surgery. Whether this rationale holds water or not depends on whether nonoperative treatments, specifically bracing, affect scoliotic curve progression at all. In short, do any cases of scoliosis exist that would have warranted surgery had they *not* been braced? Or have all bracing successes involved people whose curves would not have progressed to a degree that required surgery anyway? Since no one can predict whether or not a *specific* individual's scoliosis will progress, these questions have been the focus of a long-standing and still ongoing debate over the effectiveness of bracing. Although Chapter 3 will discuss this debate in more detail, a few words seem in order here. A recent study sponsored by the Scoliosis Research Society concluded that full-time bracing does affect the natural history of scoliotic curves: Children whose curves would otherwise have been *expected* to progress to an extent that would have required surgery managed to avoid surgery through full-time bracing. I am convinced that bracing does have an impact on curve progression, and therefore that early detection and treatment can probably eliminate the need for surgery in some patients.

Early Warning Signs

"When I was about eleven and a half, my mother noticed in family photos that one of my shoulders was higher than the other," recalls Betty, today a nurse and mother of four in her mid-fifties. "I kept making excuses, like it had to be the film or I had to be standing on a hill. It couldn't be the way I was standing. After that, my parents kept telling me, 'Stand up straight! Stand up straight!'"

Whether or not your school system has a scoliosis screening program, you can take matters into your own hands. Especially if you have any family history of scoliosis, you should not wait for the schools or your pediatrician to look for signs of scoliosis in your children. Since idiopathic scoliosis runs in families, if you have scoliosis, your children have a high risk of developing it, too. And if one of your children has scoliosis, you should be aware of the increased risk that his or her siblings will have it. Susan, who at age 45 has herself gone through four surgical procedures for scoliosis, regularly examined her daughter for any signs of scoliosis. "They didn't pick it up when they did the scoliosis screening in the schools," Susan recalls. "But I watched her back so carefully that I picked it up when her curve was only around eight degrees." If you, like Susan, are a parent who has scoliosis, be sure to inform your child's pediatrician so that the doctor knows to examine the child regularly and carefully during the course of routine physical examinations for the possible development of a curve.

You can spot some of the signs yourself, just as Susan did. Although, as mentioned earlier, parents of preteens and teens may rarely see their children naked, once or twice a year, when your child is wearing just underwear or a bathing suit, you might take advantage of the opportunity to check for asymmetry. *Asymmetry is the key to detecting scoliosis.* Although asymmetry in itself does not always indicate scoliosis, every scoliosis creates some degree of asymmetry, apparent from the front or the back. An imbalance or asymmetry noticed in the neckline, the shoulder blades, the breasts, and/or the waistline could provide a clue that your child has scoliosis. (See Figure 3.) You might also look to see whether your child's head lines up over his or her pelvis. Such improper alignment is, however, much more subtle and therefore easily missed. In addition, compensatory curves sometimes form secondary to the scoliotic curve, bringing the head and pelvis back into line.

As you examine your child, ask yourself these questions:

- Does one hip look higher than the other? Lumbar scoliosis creates asymmetry in the waist. This makes it look as though the hip on the concave side of the curve is higher than the hip on the convex side.
- Does one shoulder blade look more prominent or bigger than the other? Typically it will be the right one, indicating a right thoracic curve.
- Is the neckline uneven? Does one shoulder seem to be higher than the other?
- Do your daughter's developing breasts appear unequal in size? As a scoliotic curve develops, the accompanying rota-

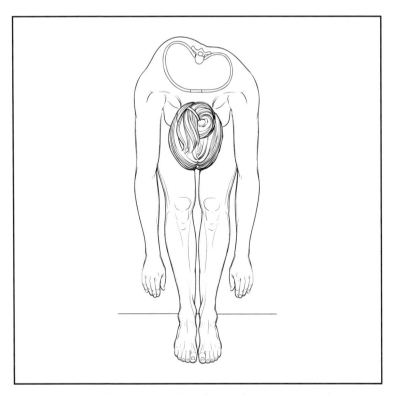

FIGURE 3. *The Adams Forward-Bend Test. This gives a tangential view of the rotational deformity of the scoliosis.*

tion of the rib cage pushes one side (typically the left) forward. This causes the breast on that side to look larger than the other breast.

If any noticeable asymmetry exists, ask your school nurse or your family physician to take a look and see what she thinks.

Despite your best efforts, however, you may not notice a curve in your child's spine until it has already reached a magnitude that requires treatment. Parents of the children I've treated often feel terribly guilty that they didn't notice the curve earlier. They blame themselves (or their child's pediatrician) for missing the small curve that has now become a large curve. It's natural to want to blame someone, but keep in mind that progression sometimes comes very quickly. During the adolescent growth spurt, a child's curve may increase by as many as five or six degrees a month! So the curve that's there now may not have been there a year ago when you or your pediatrician last checked for signs of scoliosis.

Remember also that even with early detection, no one can know what the curve progression *will be* in any individual. Predictions regarding progression are based on statistical evidence about what certain types of curves tend to do and can't be accurate for a specific patient. So even if you or your pediatrician had caught the curve earlier, the smaller curve at that stage might have indicated statistically either no treatment at all or only further observation. The curve may have reached its present magnitude anyway. So don't beat yourself up with guilt just because you didn't notice a curve until it reached 30 or 40 degrees.

Examination and Diagnosis

If a scoliosis screening test administered through the schools or by a physician suggests that you or your child might have scoliosis, you will be referred to an orthopedist for examination and consultation. Although procedures followed by individual orthopedists may vary slightly from the standard procedure described below, a typical orthopedic examination for scoliosis would proceed as follows.

Let's say that you or your child were referred to me with a suspected case of scoliosis. I would first ask a series of questions designed to provide me with your full medical and family history,
since idiopathic scoliosis is a disease that tends to run in families.
This information not only helps me make an accurate diagnosis
but also may influence the course of treatment I recommend. I
might treat a patient who has a sibling or a parent with scoliosis
a little more aggressively than I would treat someone with no
family history of the condition. Also, since the parents' level of
awareness is often much greater if they have had prior experience with scoliosis, they themselves might request more aggressive intervention aimed at halting curve progression.

I would ask about your (or your child's) birth process:
whether the delivery was vaginal or by Caesarean section, and
whether any other problems were associated with the birth. If I
was examining your daughter, I would ask if and when she had
her first menstrual period, which, along with the subsequent
physical examination, gives me an idea of her physical maturity. I also need to know about any current medical problems,
complaints, or symptoms, some of which may be associated
with scoliosis. Although adults with scoliosis may have associated back pain, most cases of adolescent idiopathic scoliosis
involve few or no complaints. A typical medical history for a
13-year-old girl with scoliosis might consist only of the information that she was the product of a full-term pregnancy and
normal delivery, that she had her first period six months ago,
and that she has no health problems, pain, or other symptoms.
Since scoliosis occurs for the most part in healthy children,
other medical problems might offer clues either that the scolio-

sis is not idiopathic or that the asymmetry is not caused by scoliosis.

Scoliosis can and does occur as a result of other medical problems, in which case it is not idiopathic. That's why we take a full medical history: to identify or to rule out primary problems that might have caused the scoliosis. A child with scoliosis who also has a history of a progressive limp and weakness in one leg is different from a child who tells me, "I feel great. I really have no problems, but the school nurse said I had scoliosis, so I have to be here." A history of bladder dysfunction may alert me to the possibility of a tumor causing the scoliotic curve. A case of polio during childhood may indicate either neuromuscular scoliosis or simply a leg-length inequality, which often presents as scoliosis because the shorter leg creates a tilt in the pelvis that resembles scoliotic asymmetry. I need to know that nothing else is going on in order to make an accurate diagnosis of idiopathic scoliosis. A complete medical history thus helps me rule out causes of scoliosis or problems that appear to be scoliosis but really *aren't*.

One of the most important indicators that scoliosis might have developed as a result of another medical problem is the presence of pain, especially in adolescents. Among children, adolescents, and even adults younger than 40 years old, idiopathic scoliosis is not typically associated with pain, rigidity, or stiffness of the spine. The presence of these symptoms in either children or younger adults serves as a warning sign that I need to consider carefully the possibility that other sources of scoliosis exist. I will try to establish or eliminate as a cause of pain a spinal-cord tumor, a bone tumor, disc herniation (this is rare), and spondylolisthesis. *Spondylolisthesis*, a fairly common condition in children, involves a slippage and separation of one vertebra from the one below, generally caused by a stress fracture of the vertebral arch. Finally, nerve-root irritation—more common among adults than children—may also cause pain and curvature that resembles scoliosis. The thorough orthopedist must rule out these other problems that may either cause or appear to be scoliosis.

THE PHYSICAL EXAMINATION

After obtaining a complete family and medical history, I begin the physical examination. Clothes can conceal the body underneath, so the patient must usually undress down to underpants for the exam. Many teenagers find it uncomfortable to undress in front of any adult—even a doctor performing a physical—and parents may want to prepare their child for the exam by explaining the procedure outlined in the pages that follow and offering reassurance as to its necessity. Most orthopedists try to be sensitive to the modesty of their preadolescent and adolescent patients, but it is likely that the child will still be embarrassed. Though some orthopedists disagree, I don't usually find it necessary for my patients to strip naked for an initial physical. If it is easier on the patient and doesn't compromise the exam, doctors should take care to respect the modesty of their young patients.

Female patients usually do need to remove their bras so the doctor can check for asymmetry in the breasts. This asymmetry may be caused by rib rotation from scoliosis and result in a deformity of the chest. If I suspect that a significant chest-wall deformity exists, I need to examine it.

With adolescent patients, I begin by assessing the degree of physical maturity. In girls, breast development, the presence of axillary (underarm) pubic hair, and menarche (the onset of the first menstrual period) provide the clearest indicators of physical maturity. In boys, the presence of axillary pubic hair, penis and gonadal development, and the appearance of facial hair signal stages of physical maturity. The degree of physical maturity is an important consideration because the risk of curve progression peaks during the adolescent growth spurt. The more mature a child is, the smaller the potential of the curve to progress. By the time a girl has her first menstrual period or a boy shaves for the first time, approximately two-thirds of the adolescent growth spurt has passed. Although these children will continue to grow, the rate of their growth and the risk of curve progression diminishes.

Next, I perform a complete orthopedic screening exam. Because I want to eliminate the possibility that the scoliosis might have arisen due to some other problem, I do not focus exclusively on the back when I perform an examination. I don't rigorously examine every joint in the body, but I do take a look at everything.

I begin by examining the way that the patient walks. Any gait disturbances might indicate some other problem (perhaps a neurological disorder or a leg-length discrepancy). If, in later measuring leg lengths, I find an inequality of more than three-fourths of an inch, I would recommend simply putting a lift under the foot of the shorter leg to level the pelvis. This may cause the scoliosis to go away.

I then perform a thorough neurological screening exam to uncover any possible neurological problems. This screening includes an examination of gait and of the strength, size, and symmetry of upper and lower extremities; a sensory exam to see whether sensation is symmetrical; a motor exam to see whether strength is symmetrical in the various muscle groups of the upper and lower extremities; and a quick check of the reflexes in the upper and lower extremities as well as the superficial abdominal reflexes to see whether they are still intact and normal or absent, diminished, or pathological. Although not constituting an in-depth neurological examination, these screening procedures detect 98 percent of neurological problems. If the results suggest that the scoliosis has a neurological origin, I send the patient to a neurologist or a pediatric neurologist.

I then examine the spine and torso, starting with an examination of the back. The key to making an accurate diagnosis of scoliosis is asymmetry. In patients who do not have scoliosis, the trunk and spine will be symmetrical. To diagnose scoliosis, I therefore do a visual evaluation of symmetry of the torso. Sitting with my eyes at the level of the back, I examine it from the top down—head, neck, shoulder heights, scapulae (shoulder blades), and waistline—looking for any signs of asymmetry or unevenness. Finally, I look at the pelvis, assessing whether it is level.

The next stage of the exam is the Adams forward-bend test (see Figure 3). While clasping the hands together, the patient bends at the waist with feet together and knees straight, bending as comfortably and easily as possible. This test allows me to see any signs of a rib hump, a prominence in the back caused by the scoliotic rotation of vertebrae.

If a rib hump exists, I measure it with a *scoliometer*. A rib hump forms as a result of vertebral rotation, making the ribs on one side of the spine rise higher than those on the other. The scoliometer, which looks somewhat like a carpenter's level, measures the degree of inclination of the rib hump. If no deformity exists, the scoliometer, which is placed across the spine at the center of the curve while the patient is in the forward-bend position, should be straight, its bubble right in the middle at 0 degrees. If a scoliotic deformity does exist, the position of the bubble on the scoliometer indicates the magnitude of the inclination. If the scoliometer tilts to 7 or more degrees, it generally suggests that the patient has a curve that may be significant. In such a case, I ask the patient to obtain a set of X-rays.

As a screening tool the scoliometer has a number of advantages: It is easy to learn and easy to use. With smaller curves, it can be used to mark curve progression without necessitating X-rays: If the results of follow-up scoliometer screening indicate an increase in the size of the rib hump, it means the curve has grown larger. Since the scoliometer measures only inclination and not rotation, however, it cannot provide an accurate measurement of the size of a scoliotic curve.

After the Adams forward-bend test and the scoliometer screening, I examine the patient from the side. During this part of the examination, I focus on sagittal curves (natural postural curves) to evaluate whether scoliosis has affected them. Thoracic kyphosis, the outward rounding of the upper back, should range from 20 to 50 degrees; lumbar lordosis, the concavity in the lower back, should range from 30 to 70 degrees. I ask the patient to bend over, allowing me to see any abnormalities that might have developed in the sagittal curvature as a result of scoliosis. Too much rounding (thoracic hyperkyphosis) or flattening (hypokyphosis) may develop in scoliosis patients. In addition, some patients with a preliminary diagnosis of scoliosis may actually have hyperkyphosis alone. Postural roundback, hyperkyphosis of muscular origin, requires no treatment other than perhaps exercise. The presence of Scheuermann's disease, thoracic hyperkyphosis that results from a growth disturbance, most commonly found in adolescent boys, may indicate the need for treatment through bracing or surgery.

Some curves look more prominent and a shift of the trunk can often be seen more easily from the front than from the back, so I also do a visual exam of the front of the body. I look for signs of asymmetry in the neckline, shoulderline, or waistline, and examine the chest for indications of chest-wall asymmetry. In girls an apparent difference in the size of the breasts might indicate that one side of the chest wall is recessed. I also check the way the arms dangle at the sides. If one elbow rests right up against the body while the other hangs farther away, it indicates that the trunk has shifted toward the side of the closer elbow. Since a high thoracic curve or cervicothoracic curve can be missed when a person is examined from behind, I have patients repeat the Adams forward-bend test while I sit in front of them.

I also check spinal mobility and flexibility by having the patient bend forward, backward, and from side to side. Children with no scoliosis or idiopathic scoliosis should demonstrate significant flexibility and mobility; adults, though considerably less supple than children, should also remain fairly flexible and mobile. Significant rigidity, particularly in children or adolescents, may indicate the presence of a nonidiopathic scoliosis.

I ask the patient to sit down to allow me to check the reflexes of the upper and lower extremities. At this time I also examine the skin for any markings, since some kinds of scoliosis are associated with skin abnormalities. For example, neurofibromatosis, also known as Von Recklinghausen's disease, or the Elephant Man's disease, which can cause scoliosis, is often associated with "café-au-lait spots," light-brown birthmarks on the skin. I also check cervical range of motion—flexion, extension, and rotation—to isolate any neck problems the patient might have. Finally, I ask patients to lie down so that I can measure their leg lengths and then conduct a quick examination of the hips, knees, and feet.

On the basis of the results of the complete medical history and physical examination I determine the necessity of future treatment. If the examination has discovered no curve or a curve of insignificant size, there is probably little to worry about, and no follow-up exams are necessary. If an idiopathic curve does exist, but measures only 3 degrees on the scoliometer and presents very little asymmetry, I suggest a follow-up visit six months later. This decision depends upon the patient's age, physical maturity, and growth potential. If the patient is only 10 or 12 years old, I would definitely ask for a return visit in a few months to monitor with the scoliometer any possible curve progression. If the patient is an adult or a physically mature 16-year-old, I would say that the scoliosis is not likely to progress or to cause any problems. Finally, if the examination has revealed a significant curve, indicated by a rib hump measuring 7 or more degrees on the scoliometer, I recommend that the patient get a set of spinal X-rays.

X-rays: Advantages and Disadvantages

Despite the risks posed by X-rays, especially to the breast tissue of young girls, large curves generally warrant a closer look that only X-rays can offer. Even a single X-ray can supply a great deal of information regarding the severity of the scoliosis and the risk that the curve will progress. An X-ray allows accurate measurement of the Cobb angle (the size of a curve), offers clear pictures of pelvic obliquity (tilt) and hip asymmetry, and provides signs of spinal maturity.

Only through X-rays can we *precisely* define a curve. Orthopedists define a scoliotic curve according to its endpoints (the vertebrae that tilt most markedly into the concavity of the curve) and its apex (the vertebra that is most rotated). (See Figure 2A–D.)

Thus, the complete definition of a scoliotic curve incorporates six elements: two endpoints, the apex, the magnitude determined by the Cobb angle, the direction of the curve, and the region of the spine in which the curve is located. A "right thoracic curve of 31 degrees from T5 to T11, with its apex at T9" means that the curve, located entirely within the thoracic spine, bends to the right, extends from the fifth to the eleventh thoracic vertebrae, and measures 31 degrees from endpoint to endpoint.

In order to measure the magnitude of the curve accurately, the orthopedist must first accurately distinguish the end vertebrae. When a series of X-rays is used to determine a curve's progression, the orthopedist *must choose the same endpoints on each X-ray.* Although this seems obvious, mistakes of this kind are a common source of error. A patient may be told that she needs surgery because her curve, which measured 35 degrees from the T5 to *T10* just six months ago, has progressed to 44 degrees from T5 to *T11* today. Yet if you went back to the first X-ray, you might find that it too measured 44 degrees if the endpoints chosen had been T5 and T11. When measured from the same set of endpoints, the curve may not have progressed at all.

X-rays also yield important information regarding a child's skeletal maturity. As children mature they develop an iliac apophysis, a separate line of bone that migrates from the side to the center of the ilium (pelvis), eventually fusing with the pelvis when growth is complete. Since a spinal X-ray always includes the pelvis, orthopedists can easily see how far the iliac apophysis, and thus, skeletal maturity, has progressed, using the Risser scale of skeletal maturity. At Risser 0, the apophysis has not yet appeared at all. At Risser 1, the line of bone has migrated up to one-fourth of the way to the median. At Risser 2, the migration has reached from one-fourth to one-half of the way to the median. Risser 3 indicates a migration between one-half and three-fourths. Risser 4 indicates migration of more than three-fourths of the distance to the median, culminating with complete fusion, sometimes called Risser 5. The Risser scale provides a much more accurate indication of skeletal maturity and therefore the risk of curve progression than either chronological age or any outer signs of physical maturity such as pubic hair or breast or penis development. In general, children who are Risser 0 and Risser 1 are very immature skeletally, while Risser 3 and Risser 4 are fairly mature, and thus there is less concern about the progression of scoliotic curves in the latter.

I generally need only one standing X-ray, preferably a 36-inch-long X-ray, which affords a full view of the spine from the base of the head to the pelvis. Although some orthopedists routinely order an additional lateral (side-view) X-ray, I find that initially an anteroposterior (A-P) X-ray—taken from front to back, with the patient facing the X-ray machine—or a posteroanterior (P-A) X-ray—taken from back to front, with the patient facing away from the machine—provides me with all the information I need to make informed diagnostic and treatment decisions. I generally ask for lateral X-rays as well only if

- the physical examination of the patient has indicated the possibility of problems with sagittal contours (kyphosis and lordosis).
- the patient complains of a lot of lower-back pain, which might indicate spondylolisthesis or some other problem better seen on a lateral X-ray of the lumbar spine.
- if I need full information on a large curve that might require surgical treatment.

Only presurgical patients (see Chapter 5) require more than two X-rays. Standard preoperative X-rays include, in addition to the standing anteroposterior (A-P) and lateral X-rays, bending X-rays, taken while the patient lies on his back and bends first to one side, then to the other. These X-rays are important presurgical tools for planning an operation—assessing where to put hooks or screws, determining exactly how many levels of vertebrae the surgeon will fuse, and deciding what degree of curve correction might be possible.

In nonsurgical cases, the only other X-ray I might order is a hand-and-wrist X-ray. No other X-ray provides as accurate an assessment of the skeletal maturity of a patient. Through analysis of thousands of hand-and-wrist X-rays, standards have been developed that allow a precise determination of skeletal age and remaining growth, which do not always correspond to the patient's chronological age. A 13-year-old may have bones that look more like a 15-year-old's, which would indicate that, though young, she has almost stopped growing. Generally, I would ask for a bone-and-wrist X-ray only if I felt uncertain as to whether a patient has enough growth remaining to make bracing the back a worthwhile option. I recently examined a 14-year-old girl who had had her first menstrual period six months earlier and had gone through a big growth spurt a year earlier. X-rays revealed that she had a 30-degree right thoracic curve and a Risser sign of 3, meaning she was somewhat mature skeletally. Since all the indications for bracing were borderline, I asked her to get a hand-and-wrist X-ray. When this showed that she had more than a year of growth remaining, I recommended a back brace in an attempt to halt further curve progression. I might also use a hand-and-wrist X-ray to help determine an appropriate time to end bracing—near the end of skeletal growth. In most cases, however, a hand-and-wrist X-ray is unnecessary.

Since the amount of X-ray exposure has been associated with an increased risk of breast cancer, many parents and teenagers express understandable concern regarding the frequency of follow-up X-rays needed to monitor curve progression. The frequency of follow-up X-rays depends upon the age and skeletal maturity of the patient. A 10-year-old child with a curve of more than 20 degrees should have X-rays taken every four months, since he has probably begun to move rapidly through the growth spurt. A 14-year-old child with the same curve, however, might need follow-up examinations and X-rays every six months, since growth has usually started to slow by this age. And a child of 16, at the end of the growth spurt, might need to return for further examination and X-rays only once a year. Adults, even those with curves as large as 50 degrees or more, might not need follow-up X-rays for two to five years, since the rate of curve progression is relatively slow in adulthood. (According to a study of adult scoliosis patients, conducted at the University of Iowa Hospitals and Clinics, the average rate of progression for all thoracic curves was about 1.2 degrees per year.) Even if you have just one X-ray taken a year, however, you might be concerned about its effects. "They took a lot of X-rays," says Betty, shaking her head. "We didn't know whether that was safe at the time, being a young girl and being exposed to X-rays as much as I was."

No one wants to do anything that might increase the risk of breast cancer, thyroid cancer, or leukemia. And frequent exposure to high amounts of X-radiation has been associated with a heightened risk of cancerous behavior in rapidly growing tissues (breast tissue, thyroid tissue, bone marrow, etc.).

Recent studies, however, have shown little or no change in the risk of breast cancer among scoliotic women exposed to multiple X-rays. A 1990 study found that the increased risk of breast cancer among this population was less than one-quarter of one percent. With proper precautions, the increase in risk should be minimal.

Of course, the most important precaution involves minimizing the number of X-rays taken and the exposure to radiation. X-rays should be taken only when appropriate—when a physical exam and scoliometer reading indicate the presence of a significant curve or when a significant curve warrants a follow-up X-ray to monitor progression. Again, I find a single A-P X-ray sufficient in most cases. Since lateral (side-view) X-rays not only require more voltage than A-P X-rays but also make it difficult to shield the breasts adequately, they multiply the exposure to the breasts, so I try to avoid ordering a lateral X-ray unless it's *really* needed.

Technological advances have also led to a dramatic reduction in the amount of radiation needed to obtain a usable X-ray. Modern equipment employs lead shields that narrow the X-ray beam, reducing radiation exposure by two to five times. A combination of high-speed film that allows shorter and shorter exposures and special filters that require less X-ray exposure to produce a picture can cut down exposure by two to six times. Reducing the amount of radiation exposure can also be accomplished through the use of breast shields, gonad shields, and thyroid shields. Both adults and children should always be provided with these lead shields, since they can reduce radiation exposure to rapidly growing tissue by three to ten times.

The final means of reducing exposure to the breasts involves positioning for the X-ray. Until recently most orthopedists took only A-P (front-to-back) X-rays, which required patients to face the X-ray beam. Today, many doctors recommend P-A (back-to-front) X-rays instead, using the body itself to block most radiation from reaching breast tissue. Although keeping the breasts farther away from radiation does reduce their exposure, the trade-off involves putting the pelvis *closer* to the radiation and increasing the exposure of bone-marrow tissue to the radiation. So the reduced risk of breast cancer may necessitate a slightly increased risk of leukemia. For this reason, I personally still rely on A-P X-rays with appropriate shielding of the breasts, although I understand why many doctors are switching to P-A X-rays.

Despite some health risks, X-rays serve as an essential diagnostic tool for advanced scoliosis. The only way to balance the necessity of using X-rays and the equal necessity of reducing cancer risk is to employ all available precautions. If, after taking a complete medical history and performing a thorough physical examination, your orthopedist has recommended one or more X-rays, discuss your questions and concerns with your doctor or the radiologist. And insist that all of the precautions discussed above be made available to you. That's your right as a patient.

Magnetic Resonance Imaging

A much-heralded way to avoid radiation exposure is magnetic resonance imaging (MRI), a technology that provides intricately detailed computer images of the inside of the body. In fact, some professionals suggest that MRIs, which use no radiation, will one day replace X-rays altogether. In general, however, I think MRIs are unwarranted and inappropriate for most scoliosis patients because they are prohibitively expensive—an MRI costs about one thousand dollars, while an X-ray costs closer to one hundred— and the information they provide is seldom more useful than that obtained through an X-ray.

In specific situations, though, where symptoms suggest the possibility of neurological dysfunction, an MRI is appropriate. A 1995 study suggests that MRIs may be warranted for scoliosis patients who have a history of severe unexplained headaches, particularly with sneezing; neck pain and stiffness with hyperextension of the neck; ataxia (a gait disturbance); foot deformities; or limited sensation of pain, temperature, or touch. If your orthopedist finds any of these symptoms during your initial physical exam, she will probably refer you to a neurologist. After conducting a thorough neurological screening, the orthopedist or neurologist might then recommend an MRI to assess the functioning of the spinal cord and nerve roots. The only other patients who should be considered as candidates for an MRI are children younger than 11 years old who have a left thoracic curve. When found in a preadolescent child, this rare curve sometimes indicates the presence of an intraspinal growth that might have caused the curve.

Generally, however, use of an MRI in scoliosis cases is a

waste of time and money. Given the high cost of the procedure and, in most scoliosis cases, the incapability of MRIs to deliver any *relevant* information not obtained more easily and inexpensively through X-rays, I see little chance that MRIs will replace X-rays of scoliotic curves in the near future.

Diagnostic Results and Treatment Options

Once the orthopedist has completed the physical examination and obtained any necessary X-rays, he and the patient need to talk about what the results mean. When you find out that you or your child has scoliosis, you will no doubt have some questions. You will want to know what effect scoliosis will have on your life, what to expect in terms of curve progression and its impact, and what treatment options, if treatment is needed, are available to you. When patients have small curves, I reassure them that they have nothing to worry about, that they don't even need to think about it for now. Most scoliosis patients, especially those with small curves, can engage in any and all activities without restriction. When patients have larger curves, however, I will spend all the time needed to answer their questions and allay their fears. Arlene, today 48 years old and the mother of four, recalls, "I asked my doctor what my recovery would be, what my chances were to have children, what my limitations would be, and physically, what I would look like if I decided to go ahead with surgery."

After learning more about scoliosis, some patients ask why

scoliosis should be treated at all. If serious medical complications and health problems arising from scoliosis have become so rare today, why would anyone need to resort to cumbersome braces or the risks of surgery? Is surgery for scoliosis merely cosmetic? In response, I generally focus on the specifics — particularly the magnitude and progression — of the individual patient's curve.

Consider the cases of a very healthy, very active woman of 40 whose lumbar curve has progressed from 45 to 63 degrees over 10 years and a 19-year-old woman with a progressive 50-degree curve. I would strongly recommend surgery for both women. Since neither woman has symptoms of pain or loss of function, they may question my recommendation. Yet curves of this type that have already become large and continue to demonstrate progression will almost always continue to get worse. Though relatively few curves progress to 90 or 100 degrees, the magnitude at which serious cardiopulmonary complications start to develop, function does deteriorate, particularly after menopause, for those with very large curves. They experience more back pain and exhibit less work and exercise tolerance. Surgery would aim to prevent curve progression and increased deformity, to help the patient avoid associated pain and diminished functional activities (work and exercise), and to promote psychosocial health. Most orthopedists would make this recommendation. Virtually all orthopedists would recommend surgically treating an adolescent with a curve of over 50 degrees or a young adult with a curve of over 60 degrees. Even smaller curves might warrant surgery if they demonstrate marked progression or if the patient complains of additional symptoms such as pain.

Surgery, of course, is not the only treatment option for patients with scoliosis. Doctors can also recommend taking a wait-and-see attitude or putting a juvenile or adolescent in a rigid back brace. The treatment your orthopedist recommends will depend on 1) the type of scoliosis you have—idiopathic, congenital, neuromuscular, or other; 2) the definition of your curve (its size and location); 3) your potential for continued physical growth (your skeletal maturity); and 4) the presence of pain, which generally occurs only in adult patients. On the basis of her diagnosis, your orthopedist might recommend any of the following:

- *Doing nothing:* If your curve measures less than 20 degrees, your risk of progression is so insignificant that no treatment is usually needed. However, a child with significant growth remaining would be asked to return for regular follow-up visits because of the heightened potential for curve progression. Unless evidence suggests progression, these visits would require only a clinical examination.

- *Continued observation.* In general, treatment isn't needed for an adolescent with a curve that measures between 20 and 30 degrees or an adult with a curve of less than 40, or even 50, degrees and no secondary symptoms such as pain. Depending on your skeletal maturity, your doctor may ask you simply to return for a follow-up exam in six months, a year, two years, or even five years if you are an adult with a moderate curve. Your curve won't progress overnight. If you are worried about the possibility of curve progression during the period between visits to your orthopedist, you can monitor progression yourself. Take photographs of yourself regularly that show any differences in curve size, rib hump, asymmetry, or posture. Also, measure your height often, since loss of height may indicate shortening of the spine due to curve progression. If these quick self-tests provide any signs of loss of height, increasing curve, or increasing rib prominence, or if you begin to experience a great deal of pain, then you should visit your orthopedist and obtain a follow-up X-ray sooner than planned.

- *Nonoperative forms of treatment:* If your child has more than a year of remaining growth potential and a curve that measures between 30 and 40 degrees (or more than 25 degrees, if 10 degrees of progression have been documented since the initial diagnosis), the orthopedist will probably recommend nonoperative treatment, specifically the use of an orthopedic brace. Nonsurgical methods of treatment will not reduce or correct the curve, but aim only to stop progression.

In the past, many different types of nonsurgical treatment have been tried. These have included exercise, chiropractic treatment, electrical stimulation, and bracing. With the exception of bracing, none of these has demonstrated any effectiveness in altering the natural history (the expected course of progression) of scoliosis.

Exercise

Although I encourage all patients to be physically active, exercise has no proven effectiveness in altering the progression of scoliosis. Exercise does have considerable value, though, in treating muscle fatigue and pain secondary to scoliosis. I will, for example, prescribe an exercise program for scoliosis patients who complain of back pain, but in such cases I would be treating the pain and not the scoliosis. I also recommend exercise to scoliosis patients who will be wearing back braces, since bracing can lead to some stiffening and atrophy of back muscles. Exercise can improve general muscle tone and fitness and help braced patients maintain their flexibility and strength. It can also increase their overall sense of well-being and self-esteem. But as a treatment for scoliosis itself, exercise has no value.

CHIROPRACTIC

Like exercise, chiropractic manipulation has demonstrated considerable value in reducing and relieving pain. Although chiropractic therapy might benefit people with back pain, I strongly disagree that such therapy can either prevent curve progression or reduce the size of the curve. Every year I see two or three new patients who have been treated unsuccessfully by a chiropractor for two or three years. Again, although chiropractic treatment can often provide pain relief, it does nothing to halt or correct curve progression. In fact, people with scoliosis who put their faith in chiropractic treatment alone may allow their curves to progress from the point where they might have been managed in a brace to the point where they require surgery.

ELECTRICAL STIMULATION

Until very recently, electrical stimulation seemed like a very appealing treatment option when compared to bracing or surgery. The treatment consists of placing electrode pads on the skin over the convex side of a scoliotic curve, through which electrical stimulation devices deliver an intermittent electric current that stimulates these muscles to contract and, theoretically, pull the spine into alignment. Although electrical stimulation can cause skin sores, discomfort, and sleep disturbances, the device appealed to teenagers because, unlike most braces, they only had to put on the electrical stimulation device at night while they were sleeping. Yet in the fifteen years that electrical stimulation has been used, no evidence suggests that it in any way changes the natural history of the disease. Statistically, the treatment's effectiveness in halting curve progression was the same as no treatment at all, and consequently electrical stimulation has now been discarded as a treatment for scoliosis.

BRACING

Back braces (discussed in detail in Chapter 3) are the only non-surgical treatment that has shown any degree of effectiveness in halting the progression of scoliotic curves. The extent of this effectiveness is still a matter of some debate. Along with the vast majority of orthopedists, however, I believe that the appropriate and timely use of back braces can halt the progression of most curves *in children and adolescents.* Keep in mind that braces aim solely to halt progression and only rarely provide any degree of permanent *correction.* Curves tend to look better and smaller while the child wears the brace, but upon removal of the brace, most curves will over time sag back to about where they started.

The Milwaukee brace, an ugly contraption that consists of a

plastic pelvic girdle, metal uprights to support the pads that push on the scoliotic curve, and a ring that circles the neck, was once the only back brace available. Today there are other options besides the cumbersome Milwaukee brace, which teenagers found unappealing and even repugnant. Many studies suggest that underarm braces might work as effectively as the Milwaukee brace. If they continue to demonstrate effectiveness, these newer braces have a distinct advantage over the Milwaukee brace: Adolescents are much more likely to wear them as prescribed. For this reason, I prescribe underarm braces almost exclusively today.

Surgery

Specific indications for surgery depend on the age of the individual patient, the location of the curve, and other factors, but there are some general guidelines. In general, surgery is warranted if the curve has continued to progress despite bracing, if the curve measures more than 40 or 45 degrees prior to skeletal maturity, if in an adult the curve exceeds 50 degrees and demonstrates continued progression, or if there is severe back pain associated with the scoliosis. Especially among adolescent patients, scoliosis surgery has proved to be safe and reliable, with a very, very low incidence of serious complications. Unlike nonoperative forms of treatment, scoliosis surgery results in curve correction. The goals of scoliosis surgery include providing a good degree of correction, stabilization of the spine in a segmental fashion, the relief of pain, and the return to a normal level of function fairly quickly.

Reacting to the News

Since idiopathic scoliosis seldom causes pain or other symptoms, the diagnosis comes as a surprise to many of my patients. Susannah, now 17, remembers how she found out she had scoliosis: "I had always felt I had a normal spine and body until I was twelve years old. I was in biology class at my school and we were assigned to do independent projects. For some reason, I chose scoliosis, just because it sounded interesting. I think I had just read a book about it by Judy Blume called *Deenie*. And I learned that one sign of scoliosis was when you noticed that one side of your skirt hem was higher than the other. And I realized that I had noticed that a lot of times. But I didn't really think much of it. Finally, I guess a few months after I turned in the report, I went to my pediatrician.

"I thought it wouldn't be too bad, that it was maybe a slight curvature. Maybe I would have to wear a brace at night. It wasn't ever going to be a big deal. I guess it was in the spring of that year, seventh grade, that I went to have an X-ray done. And I found that I had serious scoliosis. I had two curves in an S-shape. It was quite severe, a 40-degree right thoracic cure and a 43-degree left lumbar curve. And it really kind of took us by surprise. I had no idea."

Like Susannah, you may have been surprised to learn you have scoliosis. You may even have initially refused to believe it. According to one Swedish study, more than half of those told they had scoliosis initially refused to accept the diagnosis. That's one reason I spend so much time going over the results of the examination and X-rays with my patients. If you have been diagnosed as having scoliosis, it is important that you understand and accept what it means.

Of course, understanding the disease does not make everything all right. Especially among those who find out during their adolescence, when most teenagers are already painfully self-conscious, the discovery that they have a cosmetic deformity can cause embarrassment and heightened self-consciousness. Understandably, scoliosis often has a negative impact on body image. "Nothing fit right," complains Betty. "We wore uniforms and on me the dress always hung differently on one side. It just didn't look right. It was no big deal, but I knew that I was different, I knew that there was definitely something wrong with me."

A sense of belonging, of feeling part of a group, is very important to teenagers as they struggle through the confusing process of forming their own identities. Since it creates a cosmetic deformity that sets one apart from others, scoliosis can shatter a teenager's tenuous sense of belonging. Many teenagers report feeling isolated and alone during the period following diagnosis. "I didn't really know where to go or who to talk to about this, especially because I couldn't talk to family members about it," Alison, now 37, recalls with visible discomfort. "We didn't talk about it in our house. It simply didn't exist."

Whether you have just been diagnosed with scoliosis, have just picked up the back brace prescribed for you, or are preparing for scoliosis surgery, you will probably need to talk about it with someone. It could be a friend, a parent, a sibling, a psychologist, your doctor, or a member of your church or synagogue. It could even be a complete stranger. I offer to supply all of my patients with names and telephone numbers of other patients who have had similar diagnoses. Although everyone has a different experience of scoliosis, it can be very helpful to share your fears and feelings with someone who has already gone through something similar.

In talking to my patients about their scoliosis, I always end the discussion by emphasizing that *no matter how large the curve is, they can remain fully active without any restrictions other than those they place on themselves.* This is especially true of children, who tend to remain flexible and largely pain-free, despite their scoliosis. "We did know that I had scoliosis, but I had no discomfort from it," Arlene explains. "I was very athletic in high school, and I had no problems participating in any kind of sports." Only about 10 percent of those diagnosed with scoliosis ever need *any* type of intervention. So you may never need bracing or surgery. But whether your scoliosis warrants observation only, bracing, or surgery, you can still live any type of life you want to.

CHAPTER THREE

Braces: Options and Opinions

FOR OVER TWO THOUSAND YEARS, DOCTORS HAVE attempted to support, correct, or halt scoliosis through the use of external mechanical means. The ancient Greek physician Hippocrates used what he called a "forcible reduction apparatus" to attempt to correct scoliotic curves. In subsequent centuries, doctors have tried tightly wrapping scoliosis patients in bandages that held rigid splints in place, have imprisoned their backs and chests in hinged metal shells, and have encased their entire upper bodies in plaster casts. Though the modern brace has thoroughly refined and modified this ancient technique, the principles that underlie brace treatment remain the same as those set down by Hippocrates.

How Braces Work

Although braces cannot permanently correct a curve, they *can* stop the progression of a curve. Simple mechanical means straighten a scoliotic curve while it is in a brace. Pads held in place by the brace apply external pressure below the apex of the curve. These pads push on the spine, forcing it into a straighter position. The Milwaukee brace, which ushered in the modern era of brace treatment when designed by Dr. Walter Blount and Dr. Albert Schmidt in the 1940s, uses a neck ring and pelvic mold to provide traction as well. It was hoped that this "spinal tug-of-war"—pulling the upper and lower ends of the spine in opposite directions—would straighten the spine even further.

Milwaukee braces were once thought not only to act on the passive body but also to stimulate active forces in the patient. Children were taught exercises to perform in their braces so that they would pull away from the pads. Doctors would instruct children to try to be tall in the brace, to lift themselves up so that their necks rose above the neck ring. It was hoped that the combination of the brace and these exercises would stimulate and train the muscles of the upper body to pull against the curve and keep the spine straighter, even after the brace was removed. Recent studies, however, have demonstrated no increase in the activity of trunk muscles owing to bracing. Attempts to spur the patient's back muscles into taking action have little impact on the ultimate size and shape of the curve.

The constant application of force provided by the pads on a brace usually results in apparent curve correction, but this correction does not generally last. After the brace is removed, curves tend to gradually return to their original shape and magnitude. Most scoliosis patients who receive successful brace treatment thus end up no better than they began—but most end up no *worse* than when they started, either. And that is important, because the aim of bracing is not to provide permanent correction, but merely to stop the progression of the curve.

Who Should Get Braced?

Not everyone with idiopathic scoliosis is a viable candidate for bracing. The appropriateness of brace treatment depends on the individual's skeletal maturity, the size and location of the curve, and the patient's willingness to wear the brace in compliance with the doctor's instructions.

Skeletal Maturity

In general, people are candidates for bracing only if they still have at least 18 months of growth remaining, so only juveniles and adolescents should receive brace treatment for their scoliosis. A child might begin brace treatment even before he begins walking, beginning with a plaster jacket and then moving up to bracing as the infant becomes a toddler. Although such an intervention is very uncommon, some children are braced from early childhood. At the other end of childhood, if an adolescent has less than a year of growth remaining, bracing would serve little or no purpose. Since bracing is intended to halt curve progression during growth spurts, teenagers whose growth has already begun to slow would derive little benefit from a brace.

Adults have no skeletal growth remaining and should therefore not receive brace treatment *to correct or halt their scoliosis.* I do, however, sometimes prescribe a brace for older adults who suffer from severe pain but have reached an age that eliminates surgery as an option. Surgery poses too many dangers for, say, a 75-year-old woman who complains of constant and severe pain from her scoliosis, her deformity, and arthritis. In such a case, an external brace can often relieve pain simply by providing the patient with extra back support.

CURVE SIZE

In general, a child who has a curve of less than 25 degrees needs no intervention. Most orthopedists agree that children with curves that measure less than 20 degrees require no treatment at all, while curves between 20 and 29 degrees warrant further observation (every four to six months) to document any progression. Bracing is appropriate if the person's curve measures between 30 and 40 degrees. If, however, a curve has progressed more than 5 or 10 degrees, bracing might be warranted at a smaller magnitude. I would probably recommend bracing for a 25-degree curve if documented progression exists.

Curves that exceed 40 degrees prove much less amenable to brace treatment. One study found a 50 percent failure rate (meaning that the curve progressed despite bracing) among patients who had curves greater than 40 degrees treated through bracing. Consequently, patients with curves of this magnitude must, with their doctors and parents, make a decision about whether braces or surgery seem most appropriate. In the case of a 12-year-old girl who has not yet menstruated and has a

40-degree curve, I would inform her and her parents that although bracing is an option, braces fail to check the progression of curves of that magnitude 50 percent of the time. Some families will still opt for bracing, preferring to see what happens and schedule surgery only if the curve worsens; some will immediately choose surgery. Either choice is reasonable.

In a recent study, Dr. John Lonstein and Dr. Robert Winter of Minneapolis correlated curve size and skeletal maturity. Using the Risser sign and curve size as major indicators, Lonstein and Winter recommend bracing for premenarchal, skeletally immature (Risser 0 or 1) patients with curves of 25 degrees or more *whether or not progression has been documented*. Since the risk of progression is so great for this population, Lonstein and Winter argue, even if a doctor is seeing a child for the first time and cannot therefore know whether the curve has progressed, the child should be braced right away.

Although skeletal maturity and curve size serve as useful guidelines in determining who might be an appropriate candidate for brace treatment, they are not absolutely reliable, and gray areas exist. Indications become more difficult to define as a child becomes more skeletally mature. If a child had a 35-degree curve and X-rays showed a Risser sign of 4, I doubt I would brace that child. Since the child would have already virtually achieved skeletal maturity, a brace probably would not accomplish much. If the child had a Risser sign of 3 and had just had her first menstrual period, I might recommend bracing.

Other cases may seem to contradict these guidelines. Suppose an eight-year-old child had a 40-degree curve. Although a curve of this size is treated effectively with bracing only 50 percent of the time, no one wants to operate on an eight-year-old. In this case, I would recommend putting the child in a full-time brace, but I would let the child's parents know that this strategy will almost certainly only buy some time, allowing the child to mature and the spine to grow more prior to surgery. It might halt progression for a short time, but the high likelihood of progression regardless of bracing suggests the need for surgery when the child is older. If bracing fails, however, surgery would be an appropriate choice even for a young child. No child is too young to have surgery.

CURVE LOCATION

As long as the patient's skeletal maturity and curve size warrant brace treatment, most types of scoliotic curves respond well to bracing—but not all. A left thoracic curve with an apex higher than T5 or T4, and cervicothoracic curves, which are very rare, cannot be braced effectively. In the past, orthopedists and orthotists (manufacturers of braces) attempted to control these high curves through various shoulder slings and straps attached to a Milwaukee brace. But the apex of a high thoracic or cervicothoracic curve is so high that even such attachments provided little mechanical advantage. Since high curves of this kind also tend to be more cosmetically deforming than most lower curves, orthopedists tend to treat them surgically at less magnitude than they would lower curves.

COMPLIANCE

The patient's willingness to wear the brace plays a critical role in determining whether bracing is appropriate. Some kids simply will not wear a brace, regardless of whether it is a full Milwaukee brace or the more discreet underarm brace. "I wore a Milwaukee brace from the age of fourteen to sixteen," Rachel recalls, "and then I stopped wearing it just because I was starting high school and I just wasn't going to wear that thing to high school." Understandably, during this critical period of identity formation, adolescents don't like anything that sets them apart from their peers. And a brace, especially the bulky, hard-to-hide Milwaukee brace, can promote feelings of isolation and estrangement.

Clearly, the orthopedist, the child, and the parents need to consider the psychological and emotional impairment that braces can cause among teenagers. If, for instance, I have recommended a brace for a 13-year-old with a 30-degree curve and the child repeatedly insists that the brace will make him so miserable and unhappy that he'll refuse to wear it, I probably won't prescribe one. If the child will not waver from this refusal, I eventually tell parents that no matter how tough they are, they can't *make* the child wear the brace. I do not believe the physician should serve as the patient's police officer. Compliance with the bracing schedule ought to be a shared responsibility among the physician, the family, and the patient. I try hard to get patients to wear their braces through education rather than intimidation. But if a patient shows no sign of compliance, it becomes necessary to forgo the brace and go back to observing the natural history of the curve—i.e., what happens to the untreated curve. If the curve then gets worse, it gets worse. And ultimately, the curve may reach a magnitude that necessitates surgery.

Other factors do go into decisions regarding the appropriateness of bracing. Susan remembers that her own history of progressive scoliosis had an impact on the treatment of her daughter's scoliosis: "The doctor I went to would have never put her in a brace because her curve wasn't that bad, if I hadn't had scoliosis as a child." A family history of scoliosis does play a part in determining appropriate treatment. I might treat a child with such a history more aggressively than I would a child who had no family history of scoliosis. Indeed, having had personal experience of scoliosis, the parents of such children often request more aggressive interventions.

Another important consideration involves the patient's and family's feelings regarding the cosmetic deformity caused by the curve. Since brace treatment aims primarily to stop progression rather than to correct the curve that already exists, the patient must feel reasonably satisfied with the way she looks for bracing to be appropriate. Bracing will not permanently straighten a scoliotic spine, nor will it make a sizable rib hump go away. So if a patient already feels so uncomfortable or displeased with her looks that she will likely choose to have surgery at a later date, bracing makes little sense.

Contraindications for Bracing

Skeletal maturity (Risser 4 or 5), curve size (less than 25 degrees or greater than 40 degrees), curve location (high thoracic or cervicothoracic), and the patient's inability to tolerate the brace are all contraindications for the bracing of scoliotic curves. In addition, certain types of neuromuscular scoliosis probably should not be braced. For many years, children with cerebral palsy were braced, but studies now suggest that bracing accomplishes little for children with cerebral palsy. Children with neuromuscular sources of scoliosis also tend to suffer from more skin problems associated with bracing than those who have adolescent idiopathic scoliosis.

Among adolescents with idiopathic scoliosis, the only condition that might contraindicate bracing in an otherwise suitable candidate would be *lordoscoliosis*. Lordoscoliosis involves a severe flattening of the normal thoracic kyphosis, the outward rounding of the upper back. A brace may actually worsen any lordotic component of scoliosis. Since the pads used to apply pressure to straighten the curve are always placed posteriorly (from the back), they also press inward on the spine. Some degree of thoracic lordosis is a common result of bracing, so if severe lordoscoliosis already exists, I might suggest considering surgical treatment instead. Many people with moderate hypokyphosis—less than normal kyphosis in the thoracic spine—wear braces. In such cases, the orthotist should place the pads as far to the sides as possible without losing correction, resulting in less pressure on the spine.

How Well Does Bracing Work?

"I don't regret not having worn a brace in high school because I don't think it would have helped at all," Rachel says. "I just have a feeling that if I had worn it for the four years that I was supposed to, my back would have done what it was meant to do anyway."

Such skepticism regarding the effectiveness of bracing—its ability to halt, rather than permanently correct, the progression of a curve—is understandable. Teenagers hate wearing braces. Doubting their effectiveness can provide justification for discontinuing bracewear altogether—or for wearing the brace less than the 24 or 16 hours typically prescribed. It is true that in the past, some studies that demonstrated the effectiveness of bracing were seriously flawed. Some early studies that heralded high success rates for bracing failed to compare the results for braced patients with the expected outcome for patients with similar curves who went untreated. Others provided immediate evidence of success, yet failed to follow up on patients for several years after the brace had been removed. More recent and thorough evidence suggests that bracing demonstrates long-term effectiveness in the treatment of about 80 to 85 percent of patients who have curves measuring between 25 and 40 degrees, although effectiveness drops down to about 50 percent with curves that exceed 40 degrees.

Effectiveness does not mean complete correction of the curve as a result of bracing; most people braced for scoliosis should anticipate and be happy with about a 50 percent initial correction. Occasionally bracing will bring the curve of a younger adolescent with a very flexible spine down to 0 degrees. Remember, though, that this correction is rarely permanent. After the brace is removed, a curve will typically revert to its former size — but will not have increased in size. To predict long-term effectiveness in halting curve progression, braces should, within the first six months or so, reduce curves to about half of their original size when the child is actually wearing the brace. Typically, younger children with flexible curves achieve the desired reduction almost immediately simply by putting the brace on. On the first day in the brace, an X-ray taken to determine the brace's impact might show that your child's 35-degree curve now measures just 18 degrees. Sometimes it takes a little longer for the brace to reduce the curve size. The key indicator of long-term success, however, is not how long it takes for the brace to achieve this reduction, but whether or not it can maintain this reduction. If after six months, the X-ray of a braced curve shows that the curve has close to the same magnitude as it had prior to bracing, the treatment will seldom prove effective. The brace needs to hold that curve in a corrected position over the course of time.

When bracing achieves the goal of 50 percent curve reduction in the brace, the treatment has a very good chance of long-term success. If bracing does not meet that goal, the chances of the brace's working drop significantly. This does not mean that your child should immediately abandon the brace. But your orthopedist should let you know that bracing has not worked as well as he had hoped and explore possible explanations with you. Was the brace poorly made? Is the brace being worn as prescribed? Is a new brace needed?

Among patients who choose to brace curves that exceed 40 degrees, the failure to meet the goal of a 50 percent reduction over six months does suggest that bracing will not succeed in halting the progression of the curve. If a child has a curve that measures 43 degrees, and a six-month X-ray in the brace shows the curve at 38 or 35 degrees, the doctor should inform the patient right away that the brace will not work. Why keep the child in a brace for two or three more years and *then* prescribe an operation?

In order to avoid misunderstandings, patients and doctors need to review carefully each other's expectations regarding the treatment. A doctor's expectations may be quite different from the family's. The most common area of misunderstanding concerns the question, Do braces correct curves or merely halt their progression? It is important for orthopedists to explain that bracing can *only halt further progression.*

"Another reason I stopped wearing the brace," Rachel said,

"was because there was no betterment whatsoever in the degree of the curvature. It stayed exactly the same, which the doctors were telling me is good. At the same time, there's every indication that that's what it would have been regardless." Rachel misunderstood the purpose of the brace: Orthopedists do not prescribe braces with the intention of correcting a curve permanently. Long-term follow-ups suggest that, in general, if a child wears a brace until skeletal maturity and then weans himself from the brace, an X-ray taken five or ten years down the line will usually show that the curve has returned to approximately the same magnitude (within a few degrees) as it was prior to bracing. Although some exceptions do exist, the achievement of permanent curve correction through bracing is relatively rare. A responsible doctor cannot therefore promise a patient permanent curve correction that will be maintained after bracing is discontinued. Typically, if a 10-year-old child with a 30-degree curve wears a brace until age 15, the curve may drop down to 15 degrees in the brace, but will likely measure close to 30 degrees again by age 20 or so. Remember, though, that maintaining a curve at the same size represents a significant improvement over the *expected* outcome of an untreated curve of the same size. Untreated, most of these curves would progress, perhaps to a size that requires surgery or leads to medical complications.

Most orthopedists and researchers define failure of brace treatment as either a documented progression of 5 or more degrees in a braced curve or the need for surgical intervention despite bracing. Yet I'm not sure that all cases that involve either of these two alternatives deserve the label of failure. Take the example of a 10-year-old who presents with a 25-degree curve and then wears a brace until skeletal maturity. If the curve then measures 30 or even 35 degrees, should that really be considered a failure? Although the curve has progressed enough to meet the statistical definition of failure, it did not reach a magnitude that demands surgery. So I might consider it a moderate success rather than a failure. On the other hand, if a child's curve progresses from 35 degrees to 40 degrees during the course of brace treatment, that treatment has clearly failed, since the curve has progressed to a magnitude where surgery is probably indicated.

When bracing does appear to fail, the patient, the parents, and the orthopedist need to make another decision regarding what to do about it. Sarah, a small, slim girl of 15, came to my office recently for a follow-up visit. Sarah had been wearing a full-time brace for 18 months, but her curve had grown from 21 to 38 degrees during that time. Although she was postmenarchal, Sarah's X-ray showed that her Risser sign was still 0, so she still had significant growth remaining. At this stage, Sarah and her parents had three options:

1. Sarah could continue with the brace treatment. Since she still had significant growth potential, bracing remained a viable option. The treatment had not demonstrated effectiveness in her case, though. The curve had already progressed to a degree where any further progression would probably necessitate surgery. Also, since Sarah's latest X-ray had been taken after she had been out of the brace for hours rather than for a few days or a week, the immediate curve correction provided by the brace may have had a lingering impact on the shape and size of the curve at the time of the X-ray. I suggested we order a second X-ray a week later to see if the curve sagged farther in the continued absence of the brace. If this second X-ray revealed that the curve actu-

ally measured 45 to 50 degrees, Sarah would clearly need an operation. If the X-ray showed that the curve stayed the same, the family might choose to continue with the brace.

2. Sarah could discontinue bracing immediately, without waiting for the results of a second X-ray, and then wait to see what happened. If X-rays taken every four months (due to her skeletal immaturity) showed that the curve got worse, Sarah could schedule an operation in a year or two.

3. She could plan for surgery. Although Sarah's curve had not reached an excessively large degree, her cosmetic deformity was pretty bad. For this reason, she and her family might opt for surgical correction earlier.

Sarah's family chose to wait for the results of the follow-up X-ray before deciding. According to this X-ray, her curve measured 42 degrees, a borderline indicator of surgery. Considering her remaining growth potential and the nature of her deformity, Sarah and her family chose to discontinue bracing and schedule surgery a few months down the line.

How Much Do You Need to Wear Your Brace?

The amount of time a child spends in a brace may have some impact on the effectiveness of the treatment. More conservative orthopedists today still rely on the traditional recommendations for bracewear: full-time use of the brace. Full-time bracing means 22 to 23 hours a day until the adolescent has almost achieved skeletal maturity. Since most studies that have demonstrated the effectiveness of bracing in stopping the progression of scoliotic curves have involved full-time bracing regimens, many doctors still adhere to this formula.

Realistically, though, very few kids will wear their braces as much as prescribed. Although some adolescents will comply faithfully to their doctor's recommendations, many others will only pay lip service. Patients do not always tell their doctors the truth regarding how often they wear the brace. Indeed, two relatively recent studies suggest large discrepancies between what scoliosis patients tell their doctors and the amount they really wear their braces. One study compared readouts provided by transducers (sensors) built into the braces to patients' responses to their doctors' questions about bracewear. Though most patients claimed that they were wearing braces full time, the transducers showed they had actually been worn on average 65 percent of the prescribed time. In some instances the brace had been worn as little as one hour a day. Overall, only 15 percent of patients were highly compliant with the treatment protocol. The second study compared patients' responses to orthopedists' inquiries and their responses to similar questions posed by psychologists. As in the transducer study, this comparison revealed sizable discrepancies.

The question of noncompliance complicates any assessment of brace effectiveness. Very few of the studies that demonstrate the effectiveness of full-time bracing even raise the question of compliance, which calls into doubt many of their conclusions. Ironically, this undermining of the studies of brace effectiveness yields only good news for those who wear braces, because any undetected noncompliance strengthens the argument that bracing works. Patients' noncompliance may have caused these studies to *under*estimate the effectiveness of bracing. Alternatively, the effectiveness of bracing despite considerable noncompliance might suggest that part-time bracing would prove almost as effective as full-time bracing. Neil Green of Vanderbilt University, who undertook the transducer study, found no significant difference in the treatment outcomes of those who fully complied and those who only partially complied with the full-time bracing protocol.

Like a lot of practitioners today, I often use part-time bracing in an attempt to get away from the onerous aspects of full-time wear. Yet I don't believe that researchers have adequately answered the question of whether treatment regimens that call for reduced time in the brace also alter the natural history of the disease, as full-time bracing does. Short-term results seem relatively encouraging. Some studies do suggest no significant difference in results between those who wear braces 16 hours a day and those who wear them full time. (Green found 16-hour-a-day bracing effective in stabilizing curves 89 percent of the time.) Other studies suggest that 12 hours of bracing a day works well, too. Still others suggest that a "nighttime bending brace" (described in the next section), which is worn only during sleep, also seems to work pretty well. Yet all of these studies involve relatively small numbers of patients and, because they are recent, limited follow-ups. They simply don't carry the same weight in terms of numbers and follow-ups as studies on the effectiveness of full-time bracing. Until we know the results of long-term follow-up studies involving hundreds or even thousands of patients, we cannot say for certain how effectively part-time bracing halts curves.

Generally I recommend part-time bracing unless patients are at a very high risk of curve progression to the point where they'll require surgery. I would strongly advise putting a 10-year-old who has a 35-degree curve into a full-time brace. Given the child's age and the size of the curve, the scoliosis if untreated will almost definitely progress rapidly and require surgery during adolescence. My aim would be to reduce the curve size 15 to 20 degrees in one year. If at that time the child has tolerated the brace well, the treatment appears to be achieving some success, and an X-ray taken after the child has removed the brace for six hours does not show that the curve has already begun to collapse back to its original size, I might begin moving the child toward part-time bracing, perhaps 18 hours a day.

In most cases, though, I try to avoid full-time bracing because of the psychological stigma it carries and the relatively high rate of noncompliance. So with the exception of very young patients with sizable curves, I often begin treatment by trying part-time bracing first. This usually means wearing the brace 16 hours a day. The child can go to school unencumbered, but needs to put on the brace as soon as she gets home and then keep it on throughout the night. Susan recalls that her daughter "never wore the brace to school. This started in eighth grade and it really wasn't a problem until she hit about sixteen or seventeen. Then she didn't want to wear it at night when she went out with her friends."

Teenagers seem much more willing to wear braces if they can avoid wearing them to school every day. Since they tend to accept part-time bracing much more willingly than full-time bracing, I tend to give it a try at first unless the child's age and curve size rule it out. When I see a 13-year-old girl with a 30-degree curve and a Risser sign of 2 who had her first menstrual period six months earlier, I do not generally prescribe a full-time brace. Although some risk of curve progression still exists, her dwindling growth potential has lessened the risk considerably compared to that of an 11-year-old. I would probably start with a 12-hour-a-day brace or perhaps just a nighttime brace.

Orthopedists, patients, and their families should not choose part-time bracing indiscriminately. Part-time bracing should be reserved for younger children with relatively smaller curves — which might be braced a little prematurely owing to the family's concern about progression — and older children, closer to skeletal maturity, who have less risk of progression than younger kids. If in the course of regular follow-up examinations, X-rays demonstrate that the part-time protocol has not effectively stabilized the curve, the doctor and patient should then consider a shift to full-time bracing.

Bracing Options

The modern era of brace treatment began with the design of the Milwaukee brace and its widespread application in adolescent idiopathic scoliosis cases starting in 1954. Today many more bracing options are available. If you choose to undergo bracing treatment, your orthopedist may recommend one of three major kinds of braces: the Milwaukee brace, an underarm brace, or a nighttime bending brace.

The modern Milwaukee brace (see Figure 4) consists of a plastic pelvic girdle that anchors one anterior and two posterior uprights — usually metal — which extend the full length of the back and connect with a ring that goes around the neck. The pads that push on the curve are affixed almost in slinglike fashion to the sides of the posterior uprights.

Underarm braces, also called TLSOs (thoracic lumbar sacral orthoses), are sometimes referred to generically as Boston braces, after the prototype designed by Dr. John Hall and Bill Miller of the Boston Children's Hospital in the early 1970s.

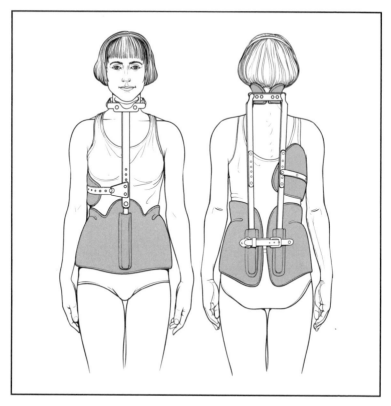

FIGURE 4. *The modern Milwaukee Brace.*

Now, however, orthopedists and their patients can choose from among a number of underarm braces, of which the Boston is only the best known. These include the Wilmington brace, European braces called the Ponte, Riviera, or the Lyon, and the Miami TLSO. All of these TLSO braces rely on the same basic mechanical principles.

Underarm braces extend from underneath the arms down to the hips (see Figure 5) and are less noticeable than the impossible-to-disguise Milwaukee braces. For this reason, most

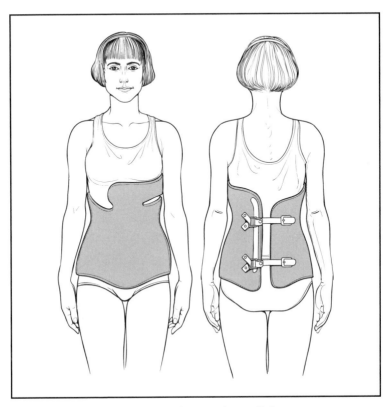

FIGURE 5. *The underarm or low-profile brace.*

teenagers find them much more appealing Although an orthotist can custom-make a TLSO, most consist of a prefabricated
plastic mold that the orthotist customizes to suit the needs of the
individual patient. The pads that push on the curve are attached
to the inside of the brace. Although underarm braces tradition-
ally opened from the rear, today's models can be front-opening
or rear-opening. The typical rear-opening brace locks the pelvis
in place, thereby reducing lordosis.

The Charleston nighttime bending brace represents the latest—and therefore the least tested—development in bracing. The mechanical principle behind the bending brace is based on observations gained from the "bending" X-ray, taken when the patient bends side to side and used to assess the flexibility of the spine and the scoliotic curve. By bending to the side opposite the concavity of a curve, a flexible, adolescent patient "straightens" the spine. If you have a right thoracic scoliosis and bend to the right, for example, your curve will become less pronounced with bending. The Charleston bending brace holds the spine in this position. Although some people can walk in the bending brace, the forced bend makes it difficult to undertake most activities. Adolescents generally strap the bending brace on every night before going to bed and wear it eight to nine hours per night.

Deciding which brace best suits your needs depends most critically upon the location of your curve and your emotional response to the notion of bracing. As the oldest and most tested of braces, the Milwaukee brace has without doubt the best track record of all braces. Researchers have accumulated much more data demonstrating the effectiveness of full-time Milwaukee bracing than they have for any other kind of brace. Unfortunately, the Milwaukee brace is also by far the least tolerable of all braces. Adolescents and preadolescents *hate* the Milwaukee brace. An unsightly and difficult brace to wear, the high Milwaukee brace sticks out above the collar line, making it impossible to hide with clothing. The nuts used to hold the slings and pads in place and affix the uprights to the pelvic girdle and neck ring frequently catch and tear clothing. Although the Milwaukee brace is a terrific tool, probably the best brace available, it's often a nightmare for children to wear. This odiousness makes it less likely that adolescents will comply with the bracing schedule recommended by the orthopedist.

Although some orthopedists still rely on them, I very rarely prescribe Milwaukee braces for scoliosis today. I use a Milwaukee brace to treat hyperkyphosis, but for scoliosis alone, underarm braces tend to work just as well for most curves. Although TLSOs (underarm braces) can effectively treat most curves, not every curve can be helped by a TLSO. In general, these braces do not work if the apex of the curve is situated higher than T7 or T6. These high curves, which account for only about 10 percent of scoliosis cases, generally require treatment with a Milwaukee brace.

I have generally had good success in treating scoliosis patients with underarm braces. Although they are no more comfortable than Milwaukee braces, underarm braces are more acceptable cosmetically because patients can hide them more easily under their clothing. Also, most underarm braces can be made more quickly and easily than other braces because the molds are usually prefabricated, which can make them less costly than other braces. Though prices vary throughout the country, in New York the cost of any of the braces discussed typically ranges from $1,400 to $2,000, which should be covered by medical insurance.

Most children find the Charleston nighttime bending brace even more acceptable than an underarm brace. Since the patient only has to wear it at night while sleeping, the bending brace has no impact whatsoever on her daily activities or social life. At first, some teenagers complain that they have trouble sleeping in it, but after a while most adjust to it very well.

The biggest disadvantage of the Charleston bending brace is that we just don't know how well it works. Several early studies suggest that it works reasonably well in treating *single thoracic curves.* The bending brace cannot effectively treat double curves because the bending that makes one curve better cannot help but make the other curve worse. One study found that after a year in the Charleston brace, only 17 percent of immature (Risser 0, 1, or 2) patients had curve progression. But these studies have involved small populations of patients and only short-term follow-ups. My own experience with Charleston bending braces has not convinced me of their effectiveness. I have prescribed a Charleston brace exclusively to treat thoracic curves, and only when patients have steadfastly refused to accept more aggressive, full-time bracing. I might also consider a nighttime bending brace if I were treating an older adolescent who might not need full-time bracing. Yet though I have prescribed very few, I've already had a couple of patients whose curves have progressed significantly while in the brace, forcing me to switch them to full-time traditional bracing. (When any part-time bracing program fails, I always prefer to try full-time bracing before even considering the question of whether surgery will be necessary.) Though some orthopedists feel very comfortable prescribing a nighttime bending brace, I would prefer to see more proof of its long-term effectiveness before prescribing it on a more widespread basis.

Getting a Brace Fitted

Far more important than the type of brace chosen is the skill of the orthotist who makes the brace. I've worked with the same orthotist for many years, because I think he does a good job. After taking an X-ray, I write a prescription for the specific type of brace chosen. The prescription indicates what kinds of pads the orthotist should use and where to put them. In a prescription for an underarm brace, I might write that the treatment is for a right thoracic curve of 31 degrees that extends from T5 to T10, and that the brace should include a right thoracic pad for the apex at T8. In addition, I always ask my patients to bring the X-ray to the fitting because that will help the orthotist know exactly what we hope to accomplish, knowledge that will help her make a better brace.

In the case of underarm braces, I have noticed little difference in the effectiveness of prefabricated braces and custom-made TLSOs. If well fitted and well made, both work effectively. Unless a patient has a particularly bad deformity that won't fit into a stock mold, I usually prescribe a prefabricated Boston brace. But if a patient or her family prefers a custom-made brace, that's fine, too.

If your child is fitted for a prefabricated brace, the orthotist will first need to measure the diameter of various portions of the trunk. On the basis of these measurements, the orthotist chooses the most appropriate stock mold, which she then customizes, cutting and trimming the brace to accommodate your child's particular size and shape and perhaps applying a heat gun to alter the shape of the brace slightly. Then she'll attach the prescribed pad or pads to the brace. Then your child will be ready for the fitting, to see whether further adjustments are needed.

To make a custom-made TLSO, the orthotist must make a perfect replica of your child's body, on which the actual brace will be molded. First, though, the orthotist marks all of your child's bony prominences so that the brace can be made more comfortable by providing some relief around these areas. The orthotist then wraps plaster around your child's bare trunk in order to make a negative mold. The orthotist carefully removes the negative plaster jacket from the trunk and fills it with liquid plaster to create a positive mold that exactly replicates your child's shape. After the inside plaster hardens, the orthotist breaks off the outer jacket; the markings that indicate bony prominences will have been transferred to the positive mold. The orthotist then constructs a brace on the mold that perfectly matches your child's body by heating a sheet of plastic in an oven and vacuum-forming it around the positive mold. Finally, the brace is cut to size and the various buckles, prescribed pads, and relief pads are attached. After a first fitting, the orthotist will make any necessary adjustments to the brace.

To make a Charleston nighttime bending brace, the orthotist follows the same procedure used to make a customized TLSO. However, before making a plaster mold of the trunk, the orthotist will ask your child to bend in the opposite direction of the primary curve in order to straighten out the spine. The plaster jacket will then be made while your child remains in this position. This allows the orthotist to create a pressure system that will push on your child's body to unbend the curve.

Like underarm braces, Milwaukee braces can be either fully customized or made from a prefabricated pelvic mold. To construct a stock-model Milwaukee brace, the orthotist will measure your child's pelvis; for a customized model, he'll create a cast, as described above. After choosing or creating the plastic pelvic section, he will contour the anterior (front) and posterior (back) metal uprights to your child's body and attach them to the pelvic girdle. The orthotist will measure the neck and select an appropriate neck ring to hold the uprights in position and stabilize the structure of the brace. Next, the orthotist will place the pressure pads on the uprights to push the spine into a corrected position. After your child tries on the brace to see how well it fits, the orthotist will make any final adjustments that are needed.

Once the brace has been made, your child will need to get yet another X-ray, this time in the brace. This establishes a baseline from which the orthopedist can later evaluate what the brace is doing. The orthopedist will also use this visit to assess the fit and check every aspect of the brace. If the brace has been improperly made or fitted, your orthopedist may order further modifications. During this initial follow-up visit I also take the time to explain to the patient and the family how and when the brace should be put on and worn, and similar details. Clearly, the process of creating the brace is uncomfortable, since it entails not only being undressed in front of unfamiliar people (particularly embarrassing for the adolescent patient), but may also involve being covered in wet plaster. As with the initial physical exam, it will probably be helpful for the child if parents explain the procedure in advance of the fitting.

Getting Used to the Brace

"It was annoying," Susan said of her experience with a Milwaukee brace. "It was a heavy metal brace; it wasn't like the braces today. It was all metal rods, and the front was like one of those old-fashioned corsets, the kind that you had to lace up and pull really tight. So it was very uncomfortable."

Whether you wear a Milwaukee brace, an underarm brace, or a nighttime bending brace, whether you wear it full time or only part time, every brace will feel uncomfortable to start. People often feel as if they're imprisoned or can't move. They complain of difficulty in breathing, eating, and sometimes sleeping. The pads built into the inside of the brace tend to cause discomfort and pain, poking, prodding, and sometimes pinching as they apply pressure to the spinal curve. Most commonly, braces lead to skin problems: rubbing, chafing, itching, rashes, and skin sores. These skin problems become especially acute during the hot summer months, since braces make the summer even hotter and typically cause wearers to sweat excessively.

"Discomfort, definitely," Rachel echoes. "And chafing. I remember you had to kind of tug and pull and do latches—it's very medieval in a way. They feel exactly like what you'd imagine them to feel like. You have a metal contraption wrapped around you. It's not pretty."

Your orthotist will address some of this initial discomfort. Braces frequently need slight modification and adjustments to make them more comfortable. But the discomfort of wearing a brace seldom completely goes away for most people. You will probably feel less discomfort as you get used to the brace, but this will take time.

Since braces do cause discomfort, I have my braced patients gradually build up to the prescribed time for wearing the brace. Imagine putting on a new pair of shoes. As you wear them more and more, the shoes will eventually give and conform to the shape of your foot. But in the beginning, they will feel tight and uncomfortable. If worn too much too fast, the shoes will cause blisters and soreness. The experience of bracewearers is exactly like this in the beginning.

Instead of telling adolescents that they must wear the brace as much as possible as soon as possible, I recommend easing into the bracing protocol. At first, you should put on the brace and wear it as long as you can, until it gets to be uncomfortable. It matters little whether the initial period lasts an hour, two hours, or just a half hour. Whatever you can tolerate is fine. When the brace becomes too uncomfortable, take it off. After the brace has been off for half an hour or an hour, put it back on. Continue to repeat this process: wearing it as long as you can, and taking it off when it gets to be miserable. Gradually, your time in the brace will get longer and longer. Through this process, almost everyone can get into the brace on the prescribed schedule within a few weeks and become reasonably comfortable with it. (As mentioned earlier, people tend to tolerate the underarm brace better, but this does not necessarily mean it's more "comfortable.") In the long run, I doubt that it makes a bit of difference whether it takes a week or a month to get used to the brace. After all, you will be wearing it for years, so a few weeks here or there should have little impact.

After wearing the brace for the first time, look at your skin underneath the brace. Your skin will most likely be red from the contact with the brace. Relieve any soreness and redness with gentle massage. Rub a little alcohol or Toughskin into the tender areas to toughen the skin and make it more resistant to chafing. A patient once told me that if you wet a tea leaf and rub it on the area, that will toughen up the skin, too. I have no idea whether this folk remedy works or not, but I share it with my patients anyway. Do *not* use lotions, creams, or powders, however, as these will soften the skin and make it *more* vulnerable to chafing and skin sores.

Since both the plastic and the pads tend to irritate the skin, you should *never* wear the brace directly on the skin. A thin, light, wrinkle-free cotton T-shirt without side seams will help reduce the irritation. During the summer, changing your undergarment frequently in hot weather to keep dry will significantly reduce chafing.

Secondary Deformities Caused by Bracing

In addition to causing discomfort, braces can sometimes lead to secondary deformities. Most of these, such as orthodontic problems, are associated only with the outmoded Milwaukee brace, and do not occur with current braces, including the modern Milwaukee brace. Braces, especially Boston braces, reduce or flatten the normal lordosis in the lower back. For this reason, most kids initially look terrible in braces; they feel miserable and look off balance because the reduced lordosis makes them pitch forward. In time, most teenagers adjust and learn how to compensate for the flattening of lordosis. Appropriate exercise aimed at lengthening tight hip flexor muscles, which also contribute to forward leaning, will help improve posture. Among those who are already hypokyphotic in the thoracic spine, posterior thoracic pads can result in a further loss of thoracic kyphosis. Often, the amount of lordosis built into a brace can be changed to deal with this problem.

Braces also sometimes make secondary or compensatory curves worse. Your orthopedist will carefully examine X-rays during your child's time in the brace to guard against this possibility. If a compensatory curve does seem to be worsening, your orthopedist and orthotist will try to modify the brace, perhaps adding additional pads, to help correct it. These alterations do not always prove effective, and in some cases patients simply have to accept the fact that their compensatory curves will get worse. However, just as spinal curves tend over time to return to their original magnitude after the brace has been removed, compensatory curves fortunately tend to improve spontaneously once the brace has been taken off.

Bracing and Physical Activities

"It was so restrictive," Rachel remembers. "I've known girls who have worn it and have been fine with it, but because of its nature, your movement is restricted somewhat and you're not allowed to do certain basic things that you had been doing. It changes the routine of your life so much that you're not going to wear it. It's too cumbersome, at least the way it was then."

As Rachel notes, braces do restrict movement. In fact, that's one of their primary functions. And this restrictiveness necessitates some adjustment in how you do certain activities. You may need to learn new ways of doing particular things that you have enjoyed doing in the past, and you may find that you can't do certain things as well as you did before. However, I know of few activities that the restrictiveness of bracing makes impossible, and for these few, I encourage my patients to take their braces off for an hour or two.

In the past—and still on occasion today—children braced for scoliosis were sometimes barred from physical education classes altogether or from certain exercises or activities in the gym. "You couldn't do a lot of the gym activities," agrees Brian, a chiropractor who spent nearly six years in a Boston brace, 23 hours a day, seven days a week. "You just didn't have the mobility and it would have been too dangerous to run around in it. I didn't develop upper-body muscle tone until I was a couple of years out of the brace."

Today, however, most restrictions on activities tend to be self-imposed. I don't restrict the activities of my braced patients at all, because I think it is extremely important to let kids feel and act as normally as they can despite the brace. If you are involved in an organized after-school sport or other physical activity—regardless of whether it's soccer or gymnastics or horse-back riding—I would urge you to participate with the brace on, if possible. If this is not possible, then remove the brace during that activity. Limit time out of the brace for specific activities to two hours, though. Some schools, because they fear injury to the child or to other children, will not let children in braces take part in such strenuous activities. So I would personally recommend that you participate in these activities *without* the brace. Take it off to swim, play baseball, Rollerblade, whatever physical activity you do after school or over the summer. Take the brace off to take part in gym class, too. The fact that you have to wear a brace most of the time should not prevent you from engaging in any activity you enjoy. You should strive to let good brace use interfere as little as possible with your life.

This recommendation to take the brace off for physical activities represents a slight departure from the standard definition of "full-time" bracing—that is, 22 or 23 hours a day. But if you add it up, the child will still spend more than 20 hours a day in the brace. And I can't imagine that those two or three hours a day out of the brace will make much difference in terms of curve progression.

Although not all braced teenagers are fully active, I believe kids can do virtually anything during the years they spend in a brace. In fact, children in braces, especially those in full-time braces, *should* exercise regularly—to keep the spine and the trunk flexible and strong. A child who wears a brace all day will clearly develop muscle weakness and stiffness. I routinely write prescriptions for a physical therapy and exercise program to complement bracing treatment. The program, fairly standard among physical therapists who treat scoliosis patients, consists of strengthening and stretching exercises for the trunk and for the legs. Again, exercise programs have no impact on curve correction itself, but play an important role in keeping the spine supple and strong.

Orthopedic Follow-ups

Unless they find the brace totally intolerable, adolescents need to wear their braces until they reach skeletal maturity. Most kids will therefore wear a brace for at least two or three years and sometimes for much longer. An eight-year-old child, whose family and orthopedist agree that bracing seems appropriate, may wear a brace for seven or eight years (as long as bracing proves successful over the first year or two and continues its effectiveness).

I generally see children frequently during the first year or so of bracing. Immediately after fitting for the brace, I will see the child to take an X-ray while he is in the brace. This gives me the chance to see whether it fits correctly and to assess the immediate correction it provides. I will often ask children to return to see me and/or the orthotist a month later, not for an X-ray, but simply to give them an opportunity to talk about wearing the brace, so that I can make sure that if they are having a problem we can quickly address it.

Your child will also need to visit the orthopedist and orthotist for periodic adjustments to the brace—or to get fitted for a new brace. If the child were not still growing, she would not be a candidate for bracing. And so the brace will need to be refitted. (The average life of a brace is about 15 months.) The frequency of adjustments depends upon the rapidity of growth.

Rapidly growing younger children might need to have their braces adjusted as often as every three months. By contrast, those who have nearly reached skeletal maturity can probably go six months between adjustments.

As your child approaches skeletal maturity, the orthopedist will begin the gradual process of weaning her off of the brace. For example, if I were treating a premenarchal 13-year-old girl with a 30-degree curve who began treatment at Risser 0, I might consider weaning after 18 months in a full-time brace. At age 15, a year postmenarchal, and now perhaps a Risser 3, her growth has begun to slow. I might ask this girl to take off her brace eight hours prior to her next visit, four months later. At that time, I'll take an X-ray to see how her spine looks after eight hours without the brace. If the X-ray shows no signs of curve deterioration over those eight hours, I will tell her that she can now spend eight hours out of the brace every day. She will finally be able to go to school without it. At the next visit, I might take an X-ray after she has spent 12 hours without the brace. If the X-ray looks good, I will increase the out-of-brace time to 12 hours a day. When she has reached Risser 4 and the risk of further curve progression has become very low, I would switch to a brace worn only while sleeping. I would not discontinue bracing completely, however, until an X-ray showed that she had nearly achieved skeletal maturity—when the iliac apophysis has almost fused with the pelvis. At that time, I will take her out of the brace and then take an X-ray after about a week or so. If the X-ray shows no significant curve progression, she could say goodbye to the brace forever.

The Psychological and Emotional Impact of Bracing

Although kids can be fully active and participate in sports and anything else while in their braces, a number of studies have shown that braces have a strongly negative psychological impact on adolescents. Whereas most scoliosis patients look back on surgery as a positive experience, almost all of those who have had to wear braces remember it as a negative experience. One study found that five of six parents of braced children described the initial bracing period as stressful. Indeed, I have found that the biggest problems teenagers tend to have with braces are psychological and emotional. They refuse to wear braces because they feel like fools and because they fear their friends will make fun of them.

Psychologically and emotionally, a brace can be very debilitating to some teenagers. Image is very important to a teenager, and my patients are always very concerned about what kind of brace they will need to wear, whether they will have to wear it outside of their clothes or under their clothes, and how much it will show. As Rachel noted, it's not pretty. However, most underarm braces can be concealed under normal, everyday clothes. "It wasn't too bad because I went to Catholic school and I wore a uniform," Susan recalls. "And with the uniform, the way it went over the brace, you really couldn't see it. So I don't think anybody really knew I had it on. It dug into me a lot and it was uncomfortable, but I don't think anybody else could see that."

The negative psychological impact of bracing and patients' concern about their appearance in the brace has already helped spark such advances as the development of low-profile braces and the increasing acceptance of part-time bracing schedules. Yet bracing still tends to heighten the already considerable self-consciousness of adolescents. Bracing, even with the more subtle underarm braces, has been associated with the development of a negative body image—though scoliosis itself has a strong negative impact on self-image. One thing that can help in this regard is talking to others who are going through a similar experience. It may be helpful to ask the orthopedist for the names and telephone numbers of other children who have similar braces. Many scoliosis organizations (see Appendix A) sponsor groups in which teenagers with scoliosis meet to discuss their problems. Knowing that they aren't the only ones and having the chance to share feelings and concerns with someone who really understands can help lessen the emotional impact of bracewear.

When first recommending brace treatment, I tell patients that, though it will take a lot of work on their part to be able to wear the brace, it's an effort they can be proud of. Kids who wear braces are helping to prevent the development of a more serious problem that may require a major operation, with all the possible risks and complications that entails. They're working hard, doing something to make themselves healthier, to make themselves better.

Finally, I tell all of my braced patients that if they just can't wear the brace, for whatever reason, it's not the end of the world. It doesn't mean they're bad people. It doesn't mean anything more than that they just can't do it. If a patient discontinues the brace and the curve gets worse, there are other options. Bracing is very difficult for teenagers. If they do it, they're accepting a great challenge, and should be proud of themselves.

CHAPTER FOUR

If Surgery

Becomes

Necessary

IF YOU HAVE A CURVE THAT EXCEEDS 50 DEGREES, a rapidly growing curve that already measures more than 40 degrees, or persistent, severe back pain associated with your scoliosis, your orthopedist will probably ask you to consider surgical treatment. The surgical procedure used to correct scoliotic curves is called a spinal fusion. The surgeon transforms a portion of the spine, which normally has many movable segments, into one unmovable piece of bone. Prior to fusing the vertebrae, the surgeon straightens the curve to the extent safely possible through the use of special metal rods. This instrumentation remains in the patient, holding the spine in place while the bone fuses. Surgery thus aims to correct the deformity, to straighten and to stabilize the spine, to prevent further deterioration, and through this correction, to relieve pain associated with scoliosis. However, before discussing the various surgical options—different kinds of instrumentation, spinal fusion, different surgical approaches, and surgical techniques—I always begin by talking to my patients about the natural history of their individual curves and explaining exactly what the indications for surgery are. So let's begin by talking about why you might consider surgery at all.

Why Operate?

What is the natural history of a curve that exceeds 50 degrees? What will happen to such a curve if it goes untreated? Most though not all curves will progress. You may already know something about the natural history of your, or your child's, scoliosis. Perhaps the curve has progressed 8 or 10 degrees in the last four years. If so, the likelihood that it will continue to progress is great. If your child is still growing, even if the curve measures as little as 40 degrees, the risk that the scoliosis will progress is equally high. In either case, your orthopedist has probably recommended surgery in order to correct and stabilize the curve.

In the growing adolescent or young adult, the indications for surgery include curve size and the failure of nonsurgical interventions (bracing). Most orthopedic surgeons recommend surgery whenever a curve exceeds a certain cutoff point. Though individual orthopedists may vary in how they define this cutoff point, virtually all will agree that a curve greater than

50 degrees in a young adolescent warrants surgical treatment. A curve that measures between 40 and 50 degrees is a gray area. In such cases recommendations for surgery depend upon the doctor's experience, discretion, and assessment of other factors (skeletal maturity, progression, deformity, etc.). Curves under 40 degrees almost never indicate the need for surgery.

"Luckily for me, I think in retrospect I probably had the best situation because they found it at a point where nothing could be done *except* the operation," recalls Susannah, whose thoracic curve measured 40 degrees and lumbar curve measured 43 degrees at the time of diagnosis, making them unbraceable, especially for a 12-year-old. "I really would have hated it if they'd found it at maybe thirty degrees and I would have had to wear a brace for five or six years. I think that would have been the worst. For the kids I know who've had the operation *after* bracing, it was this incredibly liberating experience."

The failure of bracing to halt the progression of an adolescent's curve can also indicate the need for surgery. We define brace treatment as a failure if the curve progresses more than 5 degrees during the course of treatment (see Chapter 3). Not all such failures demand surgery, however. If I brace a 13-year-old child whose curve measures 30 degrees and a year later find that her curve measures 35 degrees, I would probably not operate on that child despite the failure of bracing. I would recommend continued bracing in an attempt to prevent the curve from progressing to a degree that does necessitate surgery. If the child, especially after considering the failure of the treatment so far, won't tolerate the brace and refuses to wear it any longer, I would still not operate right away. Instead, I would continue observation, waiting to see whether the curve progresses to close to 50 degrees before recommending surgery. On the other hand, if that same child had begun bracing with a 43-degree curve and had experienced the same 5-degree progression to 48 degrees, I probably would recommend surgery right away.

In the adult, the main indications for surgical treatment consist of documented progression of a significant degree, or the presence of severe and chronic pain associated with the scoliosis. Rachel had both pain and documented progression. "I sat at a drawing table all day, and I would get backaches, but never anything major," she explains. "Then when I turned twenty-nine, for some reason I just started having really bad, chronic backaches. At first it would be after a long, strenuous day at the office. I'd go home and lie down, and it would be gone by the time I went to sleep that night. Then it just progressed so that at two in the afternoon the pain would start, and it wouldn't go away no matter what I did. And then I would wake up with the pain. And it was really, really bad for months and months.

"When you're in pain, you just want a solution to the pain. I went to chiropractors, osteopaths, and a physical therapist. Finally, I went to an orthopedist and the X-ray that he took told me that my curvature had progressed from twenty-two or twenty-three degrees when I was eighteen to forty degrees. With that kind of progression, he said that he thought that surgery might be an option."

The best way your doctor can document progression is through previous X-rays, so I would urge anyone with scoliosis to hang on to their old X-rays, as Rachel did. By comparing her teenage X-rays with her adult one, we could tell that her curve had progressed an average of nearly 2 degrees a year after she reached adulthood. Any chest X-rays taken in the past may make it unnecessary for you to wait (four to six months for adolescents, three to five years for adults) for a follow-up X-ray to document progression. If you do not have previous X-rays taken in connection with diagnosis or treatment of scoliosis, consider whether any X-rays exist from another source — perhaps an old chest X-ray taken for a job or a post-trauma X-ray taken after an accident. Any past X-ray might help your orthopedist assess progression.

Barbara, a very active 24-year-old, came into my office concerned about the possibility that her deformity, a prominent rib hump, might be getting worse. She reported no significant pain and told me that she was not aware of any progression in terms of a loss of height, or a change in the size of her rib hump or in the way she altered her clothes. She did, however, have a set of X-rays that had been taken when she was 15 years old. Comparison with a current X-ray showed a 12-degree progression of the curve from 44 to 56 degrees. The old X-rays provided incontrovertible evidence that the curve had progressed. For that reason, I advised surgery. A curve of that size would have a high risk of future progression even without evidence of past progression. Since the best predictor of future progression is past progression, her already high risk increased.

In the absence of previous X-rays, clinical indicators of progression include a loss of height and/or a change in the deformity. Patients' rib humps might get worse or they may "lose their waistline" — that is, they get short-waisted as lumbar curves get larger. Or they may notice that their hips seem further out of whack. Any of these changes provide clear indications that scoliosis has progressed.

"My scoliosis was first noticed when I was ten or twelve. It was followed for a while, and the doctor then said it wouldn't get any worse. And it did, obviously," Karin, a 41-year-old photographer, says with a laugh. "It was sixty-seven degrees when I had the surgery. It had gotten ten degrees worse in the last two years before that. We had put off the surgery because I had been trying to get pregnant. And we realized that it would just continue to get worse at that rate, which is pretty bad.

"People say, 'You were very brave,' but basically, I just felt I had no choice because of the rapid progression. I was scared stiff."

The other major indicator for scoliosis surgery in adults, chronic pain, presents its own set of diagnostic problems since the experience of pain is so subjective. The incidence of back pain in adult scoliosis is the same as that in the general population, 60 to 80 percent of whom complain of some back pain. Among those with scoliosis, however, the severity of the pain tends to be worse. "In the five years prior to surgery, I was starting to have more pain," Arlene recalls. "And getting older didn't help matters. I'm an active person, but eventually I couldn't even walk five feet without the pain. I could tell that I was bent forward as well. But my concern was to get rid of the pain, not so much the cosmetics. . . . I thought, I'm going to be fifty years old and I just couldn't see myself in a wheelchair. If I had a chance, I wanted to live out the rest of my life able to walk on my own."

If you have pain, your orthopedist will first want to evaluate whether its persistence and severity warrant surgical intervention. She will no doubt ask you a series of questions:

- How much does it hurt?
- When does it hurt?
- What activities elicit the pain?
- Are you in pain constantly or only part of the time?
- What makes the pain feel better?

- What makes the pain feel worse?
- Does the pain limit your work activity?
- Does the pain limit your recreational activity?
- What impact does your pain have on the activities of daily living?

"I knew that things were speeding up with the scoliosis. The pain was getting worse," Alison readily admits. "And I knew that my quality of life was decreasing at the same rate and eventually I was really worried that I would be in a wheelchair. That's frightening. You worry about your emotional burden on the people around you and what will happen to you. . . ."

Even if the information you provide to your orthopedist about your pain suggests that surgery might be indicated, surgery should *never* be the first choice of treatment for back pain. No orthopedist should initially treat someone who has a lot of back pain by surgically correcting scoliosis. If you have pain, your doctor will first attempt to treat it the way back pain is usually treated: with medication, with exercise, with physical therapy, with back supports. Unfortunately, the back pain of adults with scoliosis tends to be less responsive to medical management than back pain from other causes. Nonetheless, a lot of adults with scoliosis can relieve their pain simply with exercise, physical therapy, medication, or a back support.

If you have intense and recurrent (or constant) back pain associated with scoliosis and it proves unresponsive to medical management, I would advise you to consider surgery. However, the amount of pain *you* feel and the way you feel about that pain should be the decisive factor. As a surgeon, I must listen carefully to what my patients tell me and avoid imposing my values in terms of what I would find restrictive in my lifestyle. One patient told me, "I've had to restrict my activity because I get a lot of low-back pain. I don't go to work anymore. I don't go out in the evenings anymore." After hearing this, I thought that in her place I would want to do anything to relieve that pain and restore my lifestyle. But the patient said, "You know, I've adjusted to it." If the patient herself can live with the pain, it would be presumptuous of me to insist that she have an operation, that she not settle for living in such a restricted way.

On the other hand, a patient's unreasonable perception of limitation should not dictate the need for surgery. A patient who in younger days was a high-demand athlete may now find that he gets a lot of back pain whenever he plays basketball and may view this as an intolerable limitation. Yet if this is the only time the pain strikes, I would not regard that as sufficient reason for undergoing surgery. In most cases, pain that is only elicited with high-level activities should probably not be treated surgically, since the orthopedic surgeon cannot promise to get that patient back to the former level of performance anyway.

The presence of both progression and pain do not always indicate the need for surgery, at least as a first course of treatment. Sheila came to me complaining of marked curve progression and persistent but not severe back pain. Having been diagnosed with scoliosis as a teenager, Sheila brought with her more than 30 years' worth of X-rays. A comparison of these X-rays with her current ones showed that from 1962 to 1995, her thoracic curve had gradually but steadily progressed from the low 30s to the mid-60s, and her lumbar curve, from the mid-20s to the mid-60s. So she clearly had one of the two primary indicators for surgical treatment: documented progression of curves.

Sheila also had the other major indicator: persistent pain. Yet although she found the pain annoying, she did not experience it as disabling. For instance, the pain never stopped her from working. In talking with her, I learned that Sheila had never had any appropriate treatment for her pain. She had never participated in any sort of rehabilitation program, exercised appropriately, or even taken any anti-inflammatory medication. Also, she was slightly overweight, adding to the burden on her back.

Despite the progression of Sheila's curve and the presence of pain, I cautioned *against* rushing into surgery for several reasons. First of all, it would involve a very big operation. If I went ahead with surgery, I would need to perform a very long fusion from T4 down to L5, and probably a second operation to fuse the front of the spine, too. Secondly, in terms of progression, though her thoracic curve had grown 30 degrees and her lumbar curve 40 degrees, that progression had occurred over more than 30 years. Though at 46 Sheila was just beginning menopause — a time when the risk of progression may be higher — it was uncertain whether her rate of progression would change. She herself did not find her pain disabling. Finally, she was very well balanced both from front to back and from side to side, and so suffered from very little cosmetic deformity. Taking all these factors into consideration, I didn't think it was worthwhile to operate on her at that time.

Sheila may eventually need surgery, though. If her curve continues to progress in the coming years — or, more important, if her pain does not respond to other treatments and she begins to regard it as disabling — I will then operate on her. But first, I would like to see whether her pain responds to appropriate nonoperative methods. I encouraged her initially to lose some weight and to work on becoming more fit aerobically. If these do not relieve her back pain, I will still try other pain-management techniques before turning to surgery.

In addition to documented progression and pain, the question of physical appearance plays a part in the decision-making process regarding scoliosis surgery. Although appearance should never be the sole indication for surgery, I believe that any discussion of surgery as a treatment option should take appearance into account. I know many scoliosis surgeons who would disagree with me. Some orthopedists have attached a stigma to surgeons who think too much about appearance, believing that surgeons should think only about function. Granted, scoliosis surgery is *not* cosmetic surgery. But physical appearance is very important to most scoliosis patients and to discount appearance as a consideration demonstrates a lack of respect for the values and priorities of many patients.

Making the Decision

Should you have surgery or not? In making this decision, I would advise you to do three things. First, listen carefully to your doctor's recommendations and rationale. Second, ask all the questions you need to ask in order to address your own values and concerns. Finally, take all the time you need to reach a decision. In virtually all cases, scoliosis, even advanced scoliosis, is not a surgical emergency that demands instantaneous treatment. No one ever *has* to have an operation for scoliosis. If I see a 10-year-old child with a 75-degree curve, I will strongly urge that family to schedule surgery and outline all the reasons why I think the child should have an operation. Yet if the family still wants to avoid surgery, that's really their decision to make. When push comes to shove, scoliosis is *not* a ruptured appendix, a bleeding ulcer, or any other kind of surgical emergency. It does not demand treatment of any kind.

Before making any final decision regarding surgery, I would encourage all scoliosis patients to get another opinion. Any surgeon who becomes uncomfortable when you say you want to go elsewhere for a second opinion is a surgeon you don't want operating on you. You have the right to obtain all medical records as well as X-rays or copies of X-rays. So take the time to get a second opinion before you make up your mind.

In making a decision about whether to operate on a child, I would urge parents to include all but the very youngest of children in every step of this process. I like to have the kids in the room when we discuss all aspects of treatment, including very specific descriptions of the surgical procedure, what the risks are, and what complications commonly arise. Young children do not need to know every surgical detail, of course, but even with small children I go over certain basics: staying in the hospital, what to do before, giving them a feeling for what it's like to be in a hospital. Some parents understandably want to shield their children from knowledge of the specifics of surgery. But certainly by the time children reach their teens, they are almost always capable of listening and understanding—and frequently of having their own opinions, reactions, questions, and concerns. I think it really helps most kids to know exactly what's going on and what to expect. Yet if, after telling parents why I think children should participate in the decision-making process, the parents still want to avoid involving their child, I have to respect their parental prerogative.

Among children with scoliosis, deciding whether or not to have surgery seldom involves quality-of-life questions, such as the presence of pain so intense that it limits activity and the ability to function. Rather than focusing on something as immediate and tangible as chronic and intense pain, most young adults and adolescents and their parents who are considering surgery must instead focus on the uncertain future. Most of these patients are healthy and happy and functioning normally. Yet given the size of their curve, the rate of progression, and possibly the failure of bracing (if any was tried), adolescent candidates for surgery will *likely* experience problems in the future. Surgical treatment in these cases aims to prevent problems down the road.

When treating children, orthopedists rely more heavily on statistical analysis of the risk of curve progression. Take the case of a 12-year-old who has just had her first menstrual period and has a 50-degree curve. I would tell that child and her family that she should seriously consider surgical treatment. Why? Because the curve will almost definitely progress, will probably lead to pain in adulthood, and may also result in decreased functional activity and work activity as well as increased deformity and the psychosocial problems that often accompany it.

Karin recalls that when she was a teenager, her doctor offered her the option of having corrective surgery. But she and her family decided against the operation because she had also been told that the curve had stopped progressing. Now she sometimes wonders whether her family made the right decision. "Surgery for scoliosis has progressed so much in recent years that it is a plus to have had it done now," reasons Karin, who finally opted for surgery at age 38. "The way they were doing it in my teen years would have been a hard thing to go through. But if I had had the surgery earlier I wouldn't have lived with a back that was cosmetically as awful-looking for as many years — not that it's great-looking now. It's a tough call."

It *is* a tough call for adolescent patients and their families. If an adolescent, feeling happy and healthy and relatively normal, is reluctant to undergo surgery at this time, she may ask, "What's the worst thing that can happen if I don't have surgery?" The worst thing that might happen is that she will get more deformed, more crooked. If she decides later on that she *does* want surgery, it might become more difficult to do that surgery and she may not be as satisfied with the results. The rate of surgical complications also rises with the age of the patient. Nonetheless, it's still an elective decision that the family alone — after appropriate education by the surgeon — has the responsibility to make.

Among adults with scoliosis, the decision to have surgery *does* often rest on immediate quality-of-life issues. An adult with scoliosis who experiences a lot of back pain may as a result have low work tolerance or exercise tolerance and seriously diminished function. Frequently, these patients want immediate relief to improve the quality of their lives. If all other methods have failed, surgery probably does represent their best hope.

Nevertheless, if you are seriously considering scoliosis surgery because all other medical interventions have failed to relieve your back pain, you should know that no surgeon can guarantee that surgery will end your pain. The ability to relieve back pain through scoliosis surgery is not nearly as reliable as we would like. Most studies on adult scoliosis surgery have found that it provides pain relief to only about 65 to 70 percent of the patients who complained of significant back pain prior to surgery. This means that one out of three patients who undergo scoliosis surgery for pain relief will continue to experience pain after surgery. Patients must understand this prior to making an informed decision about surgery. For if they expect guaranteed pain relief and don't get it, they may end up regarding their surgeries as failures — despite any success in correcting and stabilizing their curves.

What Do You Expect from Surgery?

Patient expectations strongly influence how satisfied they will be with the results. In order to achieve a satisfactory outcome from surgery, the doctor and the patient have to have a clear and similar understanding of what can be expected from surgery. If you entertain any unreasonable expectations, then no matter what your surgeon thinks of the results, you will feel dissatisfied. But if you and your surgeon have appropriate expectations that the surgery can meet, both of you will probably end up satisfied with the outcome.

So what can you reasonably expect from surgery? The goals and expectations of surgery differ depending upon the age of the patient, the specific complaints or symptoms experienced, and the procedure performed. Since the primary objective of surgery on adolescents focuses on arresting curve progression and preventing future problems, reasonable expectations include: successful stabilization of the spine, safe correction of the deformity, a return to normal levels of activity as quickly as possible, and, after full healing, the ability to participate in all activities without restriction. Your surgeon will hope to fulfill all of these expectations. Safe correction of the deformity, however, does not mean *complete* correction. Even the most successful scoliosis surgery leaves patients with some degree of deformity.

If you are an older adult who has an established, significant deformity *and pain*, the goals of surgery should also include relief from that pain as well as prevention of any further deterioration and increase in curve size. Yet the ability to achieve pain relief through surgery, as noted earlier, varies depending on the type of curve and the specific causes of the patient's pain. No matter how successful the surgery turns out, an adult patient with low-back pain will not become completely pain-free. If things go well, the surgeon may significantly reduce your level of pain and allow you to function better, but you will probably always have some degree of back pain.

The goals of surgery also differ depending upon the specific procedure involved. Spinal fusion surgery performed from the front can generally provide better curve correction and cosmetic results than surgery performed from the back. Or if you have a thoracoplasty (see page 117), you can expect significant correction of the rib hump. Regardless of the procedure, the ultimate goal of any surgery for scoliosis is to correct the spine safely, stabilize it, and prevent it from worsening throughout the rest of your life. Cosmetic correction, though not unimportant, is a secondary concern — *to the surgeon.*

For this reason, the greatest difference between the surgeon's and the patient's expectations regarding scoliosis surgery usually falls in the area of cosmetics. I believe the vast majority of adults who decide to undergo scoliosis surgery have at least some concern about their appearance, though their primary goal is generally the reduction of pain. Some teenagers considering surgery may not care about anything other than the reduction of their rib humps and the correction of their cosmetic deformities. If I stabilize these teenagers' backs and do not correct the cosmetic deformity that is their main concern, they will not be happy with the results. For children, the risk of continued curve progression and the likelihood of future pain may seem too remote to raise concern. Despite the importance attached to cosmetic correction by most children and adults who undergo scoliosis surgery, very few actually tell their surgeon that for them, appearance is an important motivating factor.

Emily, 57, came to me with a very big curve, close to 100 degrees. After agreeing on the need for an operation, we discussed surgical options: I could perform two operations, fusing the spine from both the front and from the back, or I could operate just from the back, which would probably provide less correction. Emily insisted that she didn't care about the amount of correction at all, that she just wanted to stabilize the spine and get on with her life. I actually achieved better correction than I had anticipated and was pleased with the results. But when I showed Emily on postsurgical X-rays that her curve had been reduced from 98 degrees to just 46, she seemed disappointed: "That's the best you could do?"

Your expectations as a patient (whether revealed to the surgeon or not) will greatly influence whether you are ultimately happy with the surgery. So talk to your surgeon about appropriate goals and expectations. Make sure you understand what the surgeon wants to accomplish, why she wants to accomplish that, and how she expects to do it. Just as important, make sure you let the surgeon know in detail, prior to surgery, what *your* expectations for surgery are, too, whether they seem obvious to you or not. Your doctor will be able to tell you how realistic those expectations are. If you and your surgeon share similar expectations, you will be much less likely to be disappointed by the surgical results—and your surgeon.

Choosing the Right Surgical Team

If you have not yet found an orthopedic surgeon, or if you feel uncomfortable with your current one, don't try to find one by flipping through the Yellow Pages of your telephone book. You can take advantage of a number of resources to find a good one. If you know someone who has had scoliosis surgery, ask him what the experience was like. Find out whether he is satisfied with the surgeon and the results of the surgery. If so, you may want to contact your friend's surgeon for a consultation. Various scoliosis research groups—the Scoliosis Association of America or the National Scoliosis Foundation, for example—can put you in touch with a good surgeon in your area. (See Appendix A for the addresses and phone numbers of these organizations.)

How do you know you have the right doctor? I believe a good scoliosis surgeon must meet the following criteria:

- *Training.* Almost all spine surgeons today have been fellowship trained, as they should be. This means that after completing orthopedic residency, the doctor had an additional year of special training in spinal deformity surgery. Ask any doctor under consideration questions about his training. Did he train in spinal surgery? Did he take a fellowship in spinal surgery? If he has been in practice for more than three years, is he a board-certified orthopedic surgeon? A good scoliosis surgeon will meet all three criteria.
- *Specialization.* Before you let any surgeon operate on your spine, I would advise making sure that she specializes in spinal surgery. Personally, I don't think that doctors who do scoliosis surgery should do anything else other than spine surgery, although certainly some do. A scoliosis surgeon who also routinely operates on hips and knees and feet may lack the experience needed to perform spinal surgery skillfully. In addition, I believe all surgeons who do scoliosis surgery should be members of the Scoliosis Research Society. Ask your doctor if she is a member, and if so, for how long?

- *Experience.* A surgeon whom you allow to operate on your back should have a wealth of experience in performing scoliosis surgery. Ask your surgeon how many surgeries like yours he performs in a year. Request the names and telephone numbers of other patients who have undergone similar procedures. There's no magic number that defines how much experience is enough, but I would say that a surgeon should handle a *minimum* of 100 spinal surgery cases per year. Unless at least 25 to 50 of these are scoliosis surgeries, I would keep looking.

In addition to these criteria, you may have your own priorities in choosing a surgeon. Karin recalls why she switched orthopedists *after* deciding to go ahead with the surgery: "I had been followed by another doctor for years who had the bedside manner of a dead toad," Karin explains with a laugh. "When he started talking about surgery, I wanted to get another opinion. I had fully intended to talk to tons of doctors, but after talking to one, I really felt I didn't want to talk to anybody else. I'd never felt that comfortable with a doctor. He's as good as he is nice. And he makes you feel, when you're scared stiff, that he is the right person and knows what he's talking about. And guess what? He does."

If you consider your doctor's personality or rapport with patients an important consideration, you should take that into account in choosing a surgeon. Though bedside manner of course does not always indicate surgical skill, you need to find a surgeon whom you trust, someone with whom you feel comfortable and confident. The more your surgeon can put you at ease prior to surgery, the better the results will tend to be. Always get at least one additional opinion. Because the need for scoliosis surgery is not a medical emergency, you should take all the time you need to find just the right surgeon.

Your choice of a site for surgery is just as important as your choice of a doctor. As a rule, spinal surgery should be performed in tertiary-care hospitals (teaching hospitals) rather than community hospitals or outpost hospitals. Although not an emergency, scoliosis surgery is major surgery. It demands a tremendous investment of both people and capital in order to be performed properly. The success of your surgery depends not only on the surgeon, but on the whole surgical team. For this reason, it should almost always be done in hospitals that do a sufficient number (at least 50) of spinal fusions (though not necessarily all for scoliosis) a year. In this setting, everyone in the operating room—not just the surgeon, but the anesthesiologist, the nurses, the technicians, and the whole staff—will be familiar with the operation.

For instance, spinal-fusion surgery demands a specialized type of anesthesia. Administering the anesthesia safely and maintaining good spinal-cord monitoring requires a different type of training and experience from the kind required in, say, total hip replacements or other nonspinal surgery. Specialized anesthesiology equipment such as a spinal-cord monitor, which may cost $50,000, is also needed, as well as people dedicated and trained to operate this equipment. A spinal-cord monitoring technician, rather than the anesthesiologist, should operate the monitor. And their supervisors should also be available to help examine and evaluate the equipment if anything seems to be going wrong. As you can see from this consideration of anesthesiology, scoliosis surgery involves more than just one person. The entire surgical team should meet the same criteria of training, specialization, and experience. Teaching hospitals offer the best opportunity for medical personnel to meet these criteria.

Spinal-Fusion Surgery

When first discussing surgical procedures with my patients, I begin by describing spinal *fusion,* the major component of most scoliosis operations. In spinal fusion, the surgeon hopes to take a portion of the spine, which normally has many movable segments, and transform it into one solid piece of bone, almost like a thigh bone. I use the analogy of a fracture. If you break your arm, blood will bring new healthy cells to the area, cells that will transform into bone-forming cells. These cells lay down callus (initially just cartilage) around the fracture. This callus in turn forms immature bone within the cartilage, which eventually develops into mature bone, thereby bridging the break and restoring the continuity of bone.

I tell my patients to think of spinal fusion as a *surgical* fracture. In a fusion procedure, we strip the muscle away from the vertebrae of the spinal column and cause the bone to bleed. The body reacts to this bleeding as if it were a fracture. To heal itself, the body employs the same process described above: Cells brought by the blood lay down new bone, initially callus , which then ossifies within the cartilage, forming a solid segment of bone.

Most surgical interventions for scoliosis aim to straighten the spine or correct the curve. In some cases, however, mostly those involving congenital scoliosis, the surgeon may merely fuse the spine in its present position to prevent the curve from worsening. The goal here is not to correct the spine, but simply to stabilize it. This technique might also be appropriate for patients who experience pain related to scoliosis, but whose curves are perhaps not so large. Virtually all other interventions today, however, involve some correction of the spine.

By correcting the spinal curve and holding it in place before initiating the fusion, the surgeon can significantly reduce the size of the curve. With the targeted segment of the spine fixed in position, the new, fused bone will form and solidify in a corrected position. The segment of the spine that has been fused will no longer grow or change position. The vertebrae that once moved independently will no longer have this flexibility. In this way, your surgeon can not only achieve curve correction, but prevent future progression as well.

Bone grafts are almost always used to strengthen the healing of the spinal column in its fixed position. Bone grafting involves taking chips from another bone, usually from the back of the pelvis or from one or more of the ribs, and fusing them with the spinal segment. This mixing of old and new bone results in the formation of a stronger, more solid piece of bone.

To hold the spine in place during healing and allow the fusion to form a straighter spine, we employ a technique known as *internal fixation*. Internal fixation involves the insertion of metal hardware (*instrumentation*) around the spinal column to support it and keep it in place until the bone has completely fused. Some scoliosis patients don't understand the distinction between internal fixation and spinal fusion itself. A common misconception is that the key to long-term success lies in the instrumentation used to achieve internal fixation. Yet internal fixation merely provides the tool to obtain correction and maintain stability while the bone is healing. Until fusion has been completed, the instrumentation holds the bone in place, increasing the likelihood that it will heal in the desired position.

Once the bone heals—i.e., is fused—the patient no longer needs the instrumentation used to achieve internal fixation. The instrumentation no longer serves any function at this point, although surgery to remove it is not generally necessary. If the bone fails to heal completely, however, the instrumentation (the rods, links, hooks, screws, etc.) used for internal fixation will eventually either break or loosen. The stress of repeated bending, of the application of force to specific points on the rod again and again through everyday movement, will inevitably cause the metal to fail. If you repeatedly bend a paper clip back and forth, it will soon snap from "fatigue failure." Though the rods put in your back are a lot thicker and stronger than a paper clip, the same principle applies. The long-term success of any spinal-fusion operation thus depends not on the instrumentation but on the healing of the bone.

When they hear that spinal fusion takes normally flexible and mobile vertebrae and transforms them into one solid bone, many patients express concern about whether the operation will result in permanent stiffness. The simple answer to this question is yes. The whole purpose of the operation centers on eliminating the motion in that portion of the spine that will be fused, on fixing it in a corrected position for the rest of the patient's life. So spinal fusion always results in the loss of some mobility.

In most thoracic fusion cases, however, your surgeon will avoid fusing any part of the lumbar spine, the most important part of the spine for normal motion and function. If the surgeon can stay out of that area of the back, patients should still be able to do pretty much whatever they want after the bone heals. Obviously they will still lose *some* mobility, but not generally a significant amount of *functional* movement. People play golf, play tennis, and lift babies after scoliosis surgery. Two of my patients became professional dancers following scoliosis surgery. Others have played college football. One kid even sent me a picture of himself pole-vaulting just four months after surgery. (I would not advise this so soon after surgery. I usually tell patients to wait six months before doing any kind of activity that might entail a bad fall.)

The amount of correction a surgeon can achieve through internal fixation and spinal fusion depends upon the age, and hence the flexibility, of the patient and the surgical approach chosen. The amount of curve correction in teenagers and young adults typically ranges from 50 to 60 percent, while in adults the average is closer to 40 percent. Anterior surgery (operating on the front of the spine) can result in better correction, perhaps 70 to 80 percent in young people and around 50 percent in adults.

These, of course, represent only ballpark figures. I never tell patients what they can expect in terms of maximum or minimum curve correction. A surgeon cannot tell you with any degree of certainty how much the curve will be corrected before he gets into the operating room. During the operation itself, the surgeon will make a decision about how much he can correct the curve comfortably and safely. Knowing how much to correct is done by experience and by feel. Through extensive experience, a scoliosis surgeon develops a feeling for what can and cannot be accomplished. That's why training, specialization, and experience form the criteria for a good scoliosis surgeon. In a young, flexible patient, surgery might bring a 50-degree curve down to 10 degrees if correction happens easily and without much stress or trauma. That's an 80 percent correction. On the other hand, if the curve is very stiff, the surgeon may only be able to bring a 50-degree curve down to 40 degrees—just a 20 percent correction.

A surgeon will very rarely be able to achieve 100 percent curve correction. As scoliosis progresses it changes the shape of the vertebrae themselves. This alteration in form makes it impossible to attain a perfectly straight spine through surgery. Another reason to avoid striving for 100 percent correction is the possibility of *overcorrection.* A person who has, for example, a right thoracic curve also often has smaller compensatory curves above and below the major curve. If the surgeon performs a selective thoracic fusion (that is, fusing only the vertebrae involved in the major curve) and overcorrects that curve, the compensatory curves may not adequately correct themselves in response to the overcorrection of the thoracic region—the patient may become *decompensated.* Finally and most important, as the forces applied to achieve correction increase, the risk of damage to the spine also rises. If a surgeon pushes too hard, she might fracture one or more vertebrae or even induce some neurological dysfunction. The serious risk of these complications discourages experienced surgeons from striving for perfect correction.

Orthopedic surgeons do try to correct curves as much as they can without compromising safety. However, the primary goal of surgery for scoliosis is not curve correction, but rather balance and compensation. The ultimate objective of balance is for the head to be centered over the pelvis. To achieve balance in patients with multiple curves, the curves should be roughly symmetrical from side to side, so that one curve balances out the other one. By balancing the individual curves in this way, the surgeon can achieve compensation. Compensation is best visualized through the use of a plumb line dropped from the inion, the center of the back of the head, or from the C7 spinous process. (The bony projections at the back of the vertebrae, the spinous processes can be felt as a series of bumps down the back.) If a person is compensated, this plumb should drop down right over the center of the buttocks. If that plumb falls, say, two centimeters to the right, that person is *decompensated* two centimeters. The concept of compensation also applies to the sagittal plane (the front-to-back plane seen from the side). The orthopedist can evaluate sagittal compensation by means of an X-ray or a plumb line. If a plumb were dropped from the C7 vertebrae, it should fall just behind the sacrum. Any deviation from this indicates some degree of decompensation.

Since imbalance and decompensation affect everyday functioning much more than the magnitude of the curve itself, the scoliosis surgeon strives to preserve and/or restore balance and compensation rather than to achieve absolute curve correction. Jennifer came to see me with a 60-degree lumbar curve and a 30-degree thoracic curve. Having elected to treat just the lumbar curve, I could conceivably reduce it to 10 degrees or even to 0 degrees. Yet if I did, the surgery would create a lateral imbalance and decompensation. Instead, I asked Jennifer to have a bending X-ray taken, which showed that her thoracic curve could unbend to 20 degrees, so with surgery I aimed to correct Jennifer's lumbar curve from 60 to 20 degrees, rather than to 0 degrees. Limiting the correction of the lumbar curve to match the expected correction achieved through unbending the thoracic curve should result in better spinal balance.

Thoracoplasty

In addition to spinal fusion, the most common scoliosis surgery, orthopedic surgeons employ other surgical techniques to treat scoliosis. The most useful in terms of providing cosmetic correction is *thoracoplasty*. If you have a very prominent rib hump, your doctor may recommend this treatment. Although surgeons have performed them for many years, this technique, which can only be used to treat thoracic curves, has come much more into vogue in recent years. In a thoracoplasty, which is performed at the same time as a spinal fusion, the surgeon cuts away (resects) part of the ribs that create the rib hump (usually five or six ribs). Just prior to doing the spinal fusion, the surgeon strips the thin layer of soft tissue (the periosteum) that covers the rib to get down to the bare bone. After correcting the spine, the surgeon cuts out 4 to 5 centimeters of one or more exposed ribs. Cutting the resected rib into small pieces may yield sufficient material for bone graft to strengthen the fusion, thereby eliminating the need to strip away bone from the pelvis.

Although thoracoplasty does nothing to straighten or correct the spine, by reducing the rib hump to an average of just 30 percent of its original size it significantly improves the cosmetic result—a not unimportant consideration for many scoliosis patients. Removing sections of ribs allows them essentially to fall back into the chest, so they no longer stick out so prominently. In time, the resected ribs grow back, but the hump should not return to its presurgical size, since the deformity of the ribs results from rotation of the vertebrae. Once the spine has been properly fused, rotation should cease.

Although it can significantly improve the cosmetic result of scoliosis, thoracoplasty does have drawbacks. Since it lengthens the duration of surgery, those who undergo thoracoplasty and spinal fusion experience more blood loss than those who have only a fusion performed. It also causes more pain after surgery, particularly in the area of the rib resection. For three months or so after surgery, patients who undergo thoracoplasty will have reduced pulmonary (lung) function. One possible complication is that the covering of the chest (the pleura) may be violated as the surgeon removes a rib. Though this occurs only rarely, if it does happen, the patient will have blood in the chest cavity (a hemothorax), which can impair the expansion of the lungs. The development of a hemothorax means a chest tube has to be inserted to drain fluid out of the chest for two or three days. A hemothorax does not usually pose a serious problem, but patients should know about it in advance so that they aren't surprised if they wake up with a chest tube. Despite the slightly increased risk of pulmonary complications with thoracoplasty, adolescent patients do not develop permanent lung impairment as a result of this procedure. Adults, however, may have some slight permanent impairment. Although usually insignificant, this may be an important consideration for adults who have curves so large they already have reduced pulmonary function.

If you have a particularly bad deformity, you might want to consider having a thoracoplasty at the time of your spinal fusion. In terms of cosmetic appearance, it produces terrific results. So if appearance is one of your primary concerns, ask your doctor whether he would recommend thoracoplasty.

Instrumentation Used to Achieve Internal Fixation

"I asked to see what the rods looked like and I held them in my hands," remembers Alison. "That seems to be very unusual: to want to know what they look like, where they're going to be placed on your spine. I think all those things are important. They were to me. I'm the type of person that the more I know, the better I feel about things. There are other people who don't want to know a thing."

When I discuss spinal fusion and internal fixation with my patients, I generally do not focus on the type of instrumentation I will use. Most people have heard only of *Harrington rods*, because they have served as the standard instrumentation for nearly 40 years. Harrington instrumentation (see Figure 6) employs a quarter-inch metal rod inserted on the concave side of the curve to correct through *distraction*: pulling the ends of the curve farther apart. Hooks through which the rod passes are attached to the end vertebrae of the curve, the superior (top) hook positioned under the superior vertebra and the inferior (bottom) over the inferior vertebra. After placing the hooks, the surgeon will gradually move the superior hook up the notched distraction rod—not unlike lifting a car up on a jack. When the ends are pulled apart, the curve becomes straighter. Generally, patients must wear a postoperative brace for six months after surgery to prevent hook displacement.

Although Harrington-rod surgery is the best known surgical treatment for scoliosis, it is no longer the most common. Newer technologies introduced over the last two decades have by and large supplanted the use of Harrington rods. Harrington rods still offer the least expensive surgical alternative and have that to recommend them. This system is also by far the easiest instrumentation to insert and so requires less refined surgical skill. Yet the traditional Harrington system is almost obsolete today, used by only about 2 percent of scoliosis surgeons. Some surgeons do continue to use such modifications of the Harrington system as the Drummond system. This system further secures the Harrington rod to the spinal column through the use of a series of wires that pass through the base of the spinous process of each vertebra involved in the fusion. The Drummond system,

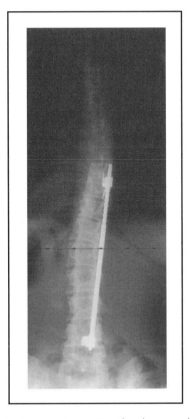

FIGURE 6. *Harrington instrumentation. Note that there are only two hooks; the rod is anchored only at the top and bottom of the curve and the rod is straight.*

which I used for many years, *is* a good system, especially for treating thoracic curves. It provides better correction and more stability than traditional Harrington rods alone, thereby eliminating the need for postoperative braces.

Though the Harrington and Drummond systems still have some applications today, the state-of-the-art technology is a segmental system, with which the surgeon can fix the instrumentation to as many points as she wants on the spine (Figures 7 and 8).

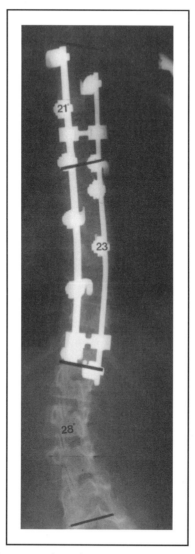

FIGURE 7. *Posterior segmental spinal instrumentation. Note that there are multiple sites of attachment of the rods to the spine. The rods are bent to create the desired spinal configuration. Several systems are available to provide segmental posterior instrumentation. These include Cotrel-Dubousset, Texas Scottish Rite Hospital (TSRH, shown), and Miami Moss Instrumentation.*

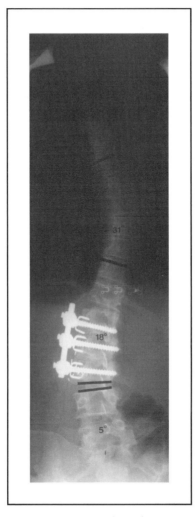

FIGURE 8. *Anterior segmental spinal instrumentation.*
This technique is appropriate for lumbar
and thoracolumbar curves (anterior TSRH shown).

The segmental systems available today go by a variety of names, including Cotrel-Dubousset, or C-D rods (the first segmental system, introduced in the 1980s), TSRH (Texas Scottish Rite Hospital), Isola, Miami Moss, and Paragon, among others. All employ the same basic principles and confer the same advantages when compared to the Harrington-rod system.

Unlike the Harrington rods, which depend exclusively upon distraction to achieve curve correction, segmental systems use a combination of forces:

- *Distraction.* Pulling the ends of the curve farther apart, not unlike the jack of a car.
- *Rod rotation.* Using the rods to derotate the vertebrae involved in a curve, turning the curve from the lateral side-to-side plane to the sagittal (front-to-back) one, thereby transforming scoliosis into either thoracic kyphosis or lumbar lordosis.
- *Apical translation.* Pulling the apex of the curve closer (but not all the way) to the midline, the straight line that might be drawn from the lowest cervical vertebra (C7) to the center of the sacrum.

Subtle differences do exist between, say, the C-D and the TSRH instrumentation. However, the similarities among all segmental systems make these differences insignificant. All segmental systems are universal—that is, they can be applied for a wide variety of spinal problems, not just scoliosis. All offer surgical flexibility, allowing the surgeon to anchor the hardware to the spine segmentally through the use of hooks, screws, or wires. All employ rods that the surgeon can contour to the spine in order to preserve sagittal curves and selectively distract, compress, translate, or derotate, whichever works best for that segment of the spine.

The advantages provided by this new wave of segmental systems include better stabilization, better correction, the ability to contour the rods to preserve or restore normal sagittal curves, better balance, stronger fixation, and higher rates of successful fusion. In addition, many segmental systems can be inserted either anteriorly (from the front of the spine) or posteriorly (from the rear of the spine), whereas Harrington rods can only be inserted posteriorly. Segmental systems work more effectively in fusing the lumbar spine than the Harrington or Drummond systems. Finally, the increased structural strength of these new segmental systems eliminates the need for postoperative casting and/or bracing, except in scoliosis cases that also involve osteoporosis or other poor bone quality.

"I had heard that when you had Harrington rods, the mobility and flexibility after the operation was very minimal and that the recuperation time was ridiculously long," says Susannah, explaining why she didn't want to have Harrington-rod surgery. "I'd spoken to kids who had to miss a year of school for it. It seemed like this drastic, unnecessary thing, and afterwards I wouldn't have a natural curve to my body—I would become like a Barbie doll, very mechanical-looking. It also seemed more dangerous in terms of so much pressure put on the one rod instead of on lots of little rods.

"When I first heard about segmental systems, it seemed incredible—something that would be able to reshape my spine to have the curve of a normal spine. I would be walking in less than a week, I would be home in less than a week and a half. I remember my mother saying, 'It seems like a calorie-free chocolate chip cookie: all the good stuff without all the fat.'"

Compared to Harrington-rod systems, the disadvantages of segmental systems are few. All segmental systems tend to be bulkier than Harrington rods. And simply because they have more hardware than Harrington systems, problems such as the prominence and discomfort of hardware under the surface of the back are more common in segmental systems. But since they have so few disadvantages and so many advantages, almost all scoliosis surgeons use one of the segmental systems today. According to a poll at a recent scoliosis conference, 98 percent of scoliosis surgeons today use some segmental system.

A typical segmental instrumentation consists of hooks (which actually look more like clamps) fixed to the posterior (rear) elements of the spine. They may be attached to the lamina (the roof of the spinal canal), the facet joints, or the transverse processes (lateral projections that provide points of attachment for muscles and ligaments). Instrumentation for a standard right thoracic scoliosis will typically employ eight hooks, four on the left side and four on the right.

To the hooks on the left (concave) side of a right thoracic curve, the surgeon will attach the first rod—usually a quarter-inch stainless steel rod. The surgeon will use tools to bend the rod, contouring it to the desired degree of correction, before inserting it into the hooks. Before tightening the rod in place, the surgeon will maneuver the rod in whatever way is needed to correct the spine—usually a derotational maneuver associated with some distraction. The surgeon then fixes the rod to the hooks by tightening down various nuts. After the left rod is secured, the rod on the right side is inserted in much the same way. Finally, the two longitudinal rods are joined together by two crosslinks, which increase the stability of the whole system.

Although they are seldom used today, three other instrumentation systems deserve mention: the Luque, the Dwyer, and the Zielke systems. The Luque (pronounced "loo-key") system introduced the concepts of segmental fixation (and therefore the elimination of postoperative braces or casts) and sagittal con-

touring of rods in the 1970s. The Luque system used two contoured L-shaped rods attached to each vertebra involved in the
fusion by sublaminar wires. Because entering the spinal canal at
every level may increase the risk of neurological damage, few
surgeons use the Luque technique to treat idiopathic scoliosis
today. Some surgeons still use the Luque system to treat people
with neuromuscular scoliosis because their bones tend to be
very fragile, making attachment of the hardware through hooks
or screws difficult.

The Dwyer system was the first widely used anterior instrumentation. The Dwyer system used vertebral screws inserted
segmentally along the curve. By placing the screws at different
levels either closer to the front or closer to the side of the spine,
threading the cable through the screw heads, and then tightening the cable to bring all the screw heads into a straight line, the
Dwyer system achieved rotational correction. Frequent complications when it was used to support thoracic fusions, a high rate
of failed fusions, and the need for postoperative bracing have
made it outmoded today.

The Zielke system operated on the same principle as the
Dwyer system, but used a thin (about one-eighth of an inch) rod
instead of the flexible cable to rotate the spine. Because it, too,
usually required postoperative bracing for three to six months,
and the rods broke more frequently than they do in other systems (though still not often), the Zielke system is seldom used
today.

Although the Luque, Dwyer, and Zielke systems—as well as
Harrington rods, of course—are still available options for surgeons and scoliosis patients, they all have limited applications
today. The safety, universality, strength, and reliability of segmental instrumentation systems has eclipsed all other systems of
internal fixation.

What the Future May Hold for Scoliosis Surgery

Segmental instrumentation *is* the latest innovation in scoliosis surgery. When Cotrel-Dubousset instrumentation first appeared in the mid-1980s it represented a dramatic departure from the way scoliosis surgery had always been performed. The whole concept of segmental fixation and derotation was radically new. Although it's hard to anticipate innovations of this kind, I know of nothing on the horizon that would have a comparable impact on the way scoliosis surgery is performed. Much of what lies ahead involves refinements of the techniques and instruments we already use today. Instrumentation will probably become a little less bulky in order to cut down on the amount of hardware and thus reduce the incidence of hardware-related problems.

An intriguing Dutch study has suggested the possibility of using "shape-memory metal" to treat scoliosis. Shape-memory metal can be bent into the shape of, say, a specific scoliotic curve and when heated above a certain "transition" temperature, gradually reverts to its original shape. Researchers hope that by "programming in" the shape of a normal spine, bending this metal to conform to an individual's curved spine, and implanting it in the back, the reversion that comes with body temperature will ease the spine back into shape. Although I find this study interesting, I believe shape-memory metal has limited applications in scoliosis treatment. It could be used only for very flexible curves. If the spine is rigid, the bone will fracture as the metal straightens out, which could lead to all kinds of potential complications, including the possibility of serious neurological damage.

In recent years, spinal surgery has incorporated various microscopic techniques, some of which may be applicable to scoliosis surgery. To remove discs in order to increase spinal flexibility and promote fusion in an anterior procedure, we currently need to perform a thoracotomy (incision in the chest wall) and remove the discs under direct vision. Microscopic techniques now allow a thoracoscopic procedure comparable to the arthroscopic surgery now commonly performed on knees. Instead of doing open surgery, the surgeon can make small holes in the chest, introduce instruments through channels (tubes) threaded through these holes, and then operate by remote control while watching the procedure on a television monitor. Some surgeons have begun performing spinal fusions using microscopic technology as well.

Yet though microscopic techniques may certainly have applications to spinal surgery, I don't see this technology replacing the techniques used in scoliosis or spinal-deformity surgery today. Even if surgeons can remove the discs and perform the fusions using thoracoscopic techniques, some sort of open surgery will still be needed to affix the instrumentation. These techniques may make some of the surgery less extensive and thus reduce surgical complications, but scoliosis patients will still need some sort of internal fixation to stabilize the spine while the bone heals. For this reason, I think any future innovations in scoliosis surgery will probably focus on modifying and improving segmental instrumentation.

The Pedicle-Screw Controversy

With the exception of Harrington rods, the only piece of surgical hardware many scoliosis patients have heard of prior to considering surgery is the pedicle screw. Owing to what I regard as an unfairly biased network television exposé, pedicle screws have achieved a certain degree of notoriety that has raised some concern among scoliosis patients. The pedicle screw is sometimes used to attach hardware to the spine by anchoring the instrumentation to the pedicle, a pillar that connects the front and back of the spine from the lamina down to the vertebral body. The screw passes through the pedicle and into the vertebral body. Surgeons in Europe have used pedicle screws for 30 years and in this country for at least a decade. Although they are available in this country and legal to use, the Food and Drug Administration (FDA), holding that the safety and effectiveness of pedicle screws have not been proved in comparison to alternative techniques, has not approved their use in spinal surgery in the United States. (The FDA will most likely approve pedicle screws for certain applications, though probably *not* scoliosis, by the time this book appears.)

Although not commonly used in this country to treat scoliosis, pedicle screws do have some value, especially in treating lumbar curves in older adults. I personally do not use them in performing scoliosis surgery on children, because children tend to have smaller curves, be more flexible, and be more amenable to simpler, less risky techniques. However, I do sometimes use them when operating on adults with more rigid, stiff curves. Since they provide very secure fixation into the bone, pedicle screws can allow the surgeon to exert more force for correction. With certain degenerative conditions, no alternative techniques exist: Either the surgeon uses pedicle screws or no instrumentation at all. In such cases, the failure rate of spinal fusion without pedicle screws would be so high that it would contraindicate performing this surgery. In most scoliosis cases, however, even if I think pedicle screws might offer the *best* alternative, I can almost always use something else.

If I were recommending to a patient the use of pedicle screws, I would first discuss what a pedicle screw is, inform the patient that the FDA has not approved their use, and explain why I think I may want to use them anyway. I would then talk about the specific risks involved in using these screws. Some concern has been raised about possible neurological injury to nerve roots as the screw enters the vertebral body. All surgical procedures, however, entail some risk of complication, and in competent hands, the risk of neurological damage due to the use of pedicle screws is low. Ultimately, I leave the decision up to the patient. If the patient consents to their use, special consent forms will need to be signed authorizing their use. If the patient does not consent to the use of pedicle screws, I understand and accept that decision. If alternatives exist for that specific case, I will use them instead. If no good alternatives exist, I will not perform the surgery.

Surgical Approaches

When talking about surgical options with my patients, rather than focusing on questions of hardware, I concentrate on possible surgical approaches. The surgeon can perform a posterior (from-the-back) fusion, an anterior (from-the-front) fusion, or a circumferential fusion (operating from both the front and the back). The choice of approach has a far greater impact on both the surgical results and the course and duration of recovery than the particular type of instrumentation used.

THE POSTERIOR APPROACH

Since almost every person who has a severe right thoracic scoliosis, the most common type of curve, will be treated with a posterior spinal fusion with internal fixation and autogenous (self-generated) bone graft, the posterior approach is used more often than any other. Selective thoracic fusions—fusing just the thoracic portion of the spine in a thoracic curve that has led to the development of a compensatory lumbar curve—are almost always performed posteriorly. Fusions of double major curves (comparably large thoracic and lumbar curves) are also generally done from behind.

In a posterior procedure, the surgeon will first make an incision that runs down the middle of the back. The length of this incision depends on the length of the spinal fusion. After stripping away all the muscle to get down to the bare bone, the surgeon will resect (surgically remove) all the facet joints in the area of the spine targeted for fusion. This resection improves the flexibility of the spine and allows for better correction. The surgeon next applies the instruments, the hooks and rods, to the spine and uses them to obtain the desired degree of correction. Then she roughens and strips away the outer surface of the bone, causing it to bleed. The surgeon will have obtained material for bone graft, chips of bone taken either from the ilium (the back of the pelvis) or from the ribs if a thoracoplasty is also being performed. After putting in those chips of bone, the surgeon closes the muscle and stitches up the skin.

THE ANTERIOR APPROACH

The anterior approach means operating on the spine from the front. Although some surgeons will fuse thoracic curves from the front, most surgeons in this country employ this approach primarily in treating lumbar and thoracolumbar curves, curves with an apex situated on the thoracolumbar juncture. Especially when treating teenagers and young adults with these kinds of curves, I consider it the procedure of choice. By operating on these curves from the front, the surgeon can do much shorter fusions, while at the same time getting better correction. Since the lumbar spine plays a critical role in everyday mobility, shorter fusions in this area provide a big advantage, allowing the surgeon to preserve more motion segments—parts of the spine that still afford mobility—and thus prevent excessive stiffening and loss of mobility. In addition, the lower down in the lumbar spine a fusion goes, the greater the risk that the patient will eventually develop back pain as a consequence of surgery. So if I can perform a shorter fusion by using an anterior approach and thus avoid fusing the spine below L2 or L3, I can significantly reduce the risk that my patient will later experience back pain.

In an anterior procedure, the surgeon begins by making an incision in the patient's *side*, not the front, and then continues the incision down and to the front. To get to the spine, the surgeon removes one of the ribs and uses it as material for bone graft. In most anterior procedures, the surgeon then takes out all of the discs through the length of the spine that will be fused. Removal of the discs creates greater spinal mobility and flexibility and creates a broader area for fusion by putting bone on bone where the discs once separated the vertebrae. Removal of the discs also facilitates compression. By taking out the discs, the surgeon can compress the convex side of the curve and get some correction that way. The surgeon then installs the instrumentation, prepares the bone for grafting, and puts in the material obtained from the rib before closing the incision.

C O M B I N E D   A N T E R I O R   A N D

P O S T E R I O R   A P P R O A C H E S

A patient who has a very large and very rigid curve — one measuring more than 75 or 80 degrees on a *bending* X-ray — will probably achieve the best results by undergoing both anterior and posterior procedures (A/P surgery). If a patient's standing X-ray revealed a 75-degree thoracic curve, and that person's bending X-ray was also 75 degrees, I'd know that person has no flexibility in his or her spine. If, on the other hand, the bending X-ray showed that bending brings the curve down to only 40 degrees, I would probably not see the need to operate on that person from the front. A/P surgery can create additional flexibility while providing better correction, additional stabilization, and a higher rate of fusion. Most of the correction would be achieved through posterior surgery, while the anterior procedure would promote increased flexibility for the posterior correction and also provide more area for fusion. In some cases, anterior instrumentation may also be used. As adults grow older, the rate of *pseudoarthrosis* — the failure of fusion — increases. By operating front and back, performing a circumferential (wrap-around) fusion, the surgeon can considerably reduce that pseudoarthrosis rate.

Where does the line fall that makes the anterior/posterior

approach preferable to only anterior or posterior surgery? It's partly arbitrary, depending upon the experience and feeling of the surgeon. I usually recommend stabilizing lumbar curves from the back as well as the front once a patient passes the age of 40. Although the posterior surgery does not provide any additional correction, it further stabilizes the curve, which becomes more important as the risk of pseudoarthrosis increases.

A/P surgery is also appropriate for patients who have significant sagittal-plane problems. If you have lost a lot of lordosis and have developed sagittal balance problems, your surgeon may need to build up the front of your spine to correct not only the lateral scoliotic curve but also the sagittal curves. By lengthening the spine in the front but maintaining the length of the spine in the back, the surgeon can induce more appropriate sagittal curves. If you have excessive thoracic kyphosis, the surgeon will also need to operate on the kyphotic portion of the curve from the front as well as the back. Finally, certain diagnoses such as neuromuscular scolioses (e.g., cerebral palsy and scoliosis) require front and back surgery.

Anterior and posterior surgery is rarely used in operating on children, who generally have smaller, more flexible curves. However, if a child is very young, say, under the age of 10 or 11, I would strongly consider A/P surgery. The need for surgery in such young children is more common with congenital scoliosis and rarely occurs with idiopathic scoliosis. In such cases, A/P surgery is recommended to prevent the significant risk that the child will develop a postoperative condition known as the "crankshaft phenomenon." When a young child has only a posterior segment of his or her spine fused, the front of the spine will continue to grow as the child matures. Yet since fusion has tethered the posterior spine, preventing it from lengthening, the growing spine rotates like the crankshaft of a car, with the front bending back and forth. As a consequence, despite the posterior fusion, the child's deformity increases. In such cases, the surgeon needs to supplement posterior fusion with anterior fusion to prevent this phenomenon. This essentially arrests growth in the fused segment of the spine.

In most A/P surgery today, anterior and posterior procedures are performed under one anesthesia. This makes A/P surgery an exceedingly long procedure, requiring perhaps 8, 10, or even 12 hours in the operating room. "I think it was a lot to go through the front and the back at the same time," says Arlene, who underwent A/P surgery. "But the surgeon knew I was a gutsy woman and I said to him, 'Let's do it in one shot.' 'Cause I didn't know if I'd go back."

The procedures follow essentially the same course described above for the anterior and posterior approaches. The length of surgery, however, raises some concern with many patients, who want to know whether it's safe for them to have that much anesthesia. Actually, it's safer, since patients receive less total anesthesia by having both procedures done at once than they would if the procedures were separated. They also have significantly less blood loss and much shorter hospitalizations.

Patients who undergo A/P surgery do not necessarily require instrumentation in both the front and back of the spine. A lot of scoliosis surgeons will perform just releases (the removal of discs to untether the spine and provide greater flexibility for correction) and fusions anteriorly, and then instrument only from the back. When I treat lumbar curves with A/P surgery, though, I tend to instrument from the front as well as the back. I believe that instrumentation from the front allows me to get better correction and better stabilization, making it easier then to instrument from the back.

As Arlene acknowledges, undergoing A/P surgery is a lot to go through. When recommending combined posterior and anterior approaches, I carefully outline my rationale to patients. But not every patient wants to go through such extensive surgery. Sometimes a person tells me, "Look, I don't care that you can get better correction if you operate on me from the front as well. It's not that important to me. I'm willing to accept the increased rate of failure, because if it fails you can always redo it and fix it at that point. But for now, just do me from the back. It's simpler and easier and I'll get back to my life more quickly." In most such cases, I consent to the patient's wishes. Although I may think A/P surgery is *better* than anterior only or posterior only, in most cases it would not be wrong to operate only from the front or the back. (Certain cases do require A/P surgery in order to achieve appropriate balance.) So though I will make specific recommendations, I generally leave the final decision up to the patient.

Possible Surgical Complications

Every surgical procedure carries with it the risk of complications, and patients making decisions about surgery have a right to know about any potential risks. To be fair with my patients, I outline as explicitly as possible the complications that might arise from the surgery, for two reasons. First, the patient needs this information to make fully informed decisions about whether to have surgery and about what procedure the doctor should use. Also, I find that this information helps patients cope better with any complications that do arise after surgery. Certainly I don't cover every potential complication, because that would be impossible. But I do try to talk clearly about the things that happen most commonly (pseudoarthrosis, problems with rods or other hardware, medical complications such as pneumonia) and about the things that patients tend to be most concerned about, such as neurological damage.

Any surgical complications are possible, so I don't want to underemphasize them, but all complications need to be put into perspective. For otherwise healthy kids and young adults, scoliosis surgery is absolutely straightforward and reliable 97 or 98 times out of 100. The vast majority of younger patients with scoliosis check into the hospital, have their surgery, and leave a week later without any particular problems. The complication rate from surgery does rise as people grow older. Among adults, the complication rate from scoliosis surgery ranges anywhere from 35 to 70 percent. Although this seems like a lot, most of these complications are minor and can be resolved with appropriate treatment.

The complication that most concerns people facing scoliosis surgery is the possibility of neurological damage. Any operation on the spinal column carries the risk of injury to the spinal cord or nerve roots. Although rare (occurring in less than 1 percent of all scoliosis operations), a wide range of neurological injuries are possible as a result of scoliosis surgery. The worst possible neurological injury would involve some degree of paralysis. Injury to the spinal cord could leave you unable to move your legs or perhaps unable to control your bowel and bladder functions. I do discuss paralysis as a worst-case scenario, but I reassure my patients that scoliosis surgery has never caused paralysis in any of my patients to date.

Other possible neurological problems include a range of partial spinal-cord injuries. Brown-Sequard syndrome involves injury to one-half of the spinal cord, resulting in a sensory deficit on one side of the body and a motor deficit on the other side. These partial cord lesions usually recover on their own. A nerve-root injury, damage to one specific nerve root, might interfere with the ability to move or control a specific muscle. Minor neurological injuries might also cause a specific distribution of pain or such sensory problems as numbness and tingling. Very few of these injuries to the spinal cord result from a direct blow—for example, an instrument that slips. Instead, most are vascular in nature, stemming from some local interference with the segmental blood supply to the spinal cord.

Though scoliosis surgery *can* result in any of these neurological injuries, very, very few operations actually cause them. Scoliosis surgeons recognize the risks involved in operating so close to the spinal cord, and do everything possible to guard against neurological damage. During the operation itself, sophisticated spinal-cord monitors keep track of neurological functioning throughout the spinal cord. Many surgeons also use a "wake-up" test, which involves bringing the patient up from the anesthesia and asking her to wiggle her toes in order to demonstrate normal neurological functioning. Finally, one of the reasons surgeons do not try to overcorrect scoliotic curves—for example, bringing a 70-degree curve down to 10 degrees—is to avoid neurological injuries. Instead, surgeons try to achieve *reasonable* correction that protects the safety of the patient.

Of the other possible complications, none poses the kind of threat that neurological damage does. The most common complications are pseudoarthrosis (the failure of the bone to fuse), hardware complications (the breaking or loosening of instrumentation), and problems involving the prominence and painfulness of hardware. Any of these problems may entail further surgery, either to promote fusion or to remove the hardware. Although relatively rare, some patients complain of persistent pain from the site of the bone graft. Everyone experiences pain at the graft site, but normally it goes away with time.

Instrumentation systems that achieve curve correction chiefly through distraction, such as Harrington rods, carry the significant risk of creating a "flat back." Pulling the ends of the curve farther apart can reduce not only the lateral scoliotic curve but also the normal sagittal curves. This can result in the loss of lumbar lordosis, or a flattening of the lower back. Contoured rods and compression techniques can help preserve lordosis and avoid this complication. (Compressing—reducing the length of—the posterior portion of the lumbar spine causes the anterior portion, which retains its original size, to arch backward, thereby preserving or restoring lordosis.)

Finally, as with any surgery, patients may also develop medical problems from scoliosis surgery. The most common of these are pneumonia, infection, cardiac arrhythmia, ileus (a bowel dysfunction that causes the belly to become distended), and urinary-tract infections, a result of the Foley catheter. Although other complications are rare, virtually any normal surgical complication is possible.

Whether you have anterior or posterior surgery will not affect the risk of complication, although certain complications are more common with one approach than the other. The frequency of pulmonary complications is higher using an anterior approach. Operating from the front also carries the risk of putting a hole in one of the great blood vessels, such as the aorta, which cannot happen with posterior procedures. Anterior surgery on males with scoliosis also entails a small risk (0.5 to 1 percent) of retrograde ejaculation: The man remains potent and capable of erection, but the semen, instead of ejaculating, backs up. This condition may correct itself. (The one patient I've seen who had retrograde ejaculation recovered spontaneously.) Finally, an ileus, or bowel obstruction, occurs more commonly after anterior procedures than posterior ones. On the other hand, posterior approaches to scoliosis surgery generally involve a higher blood loss. Posterior instrumentation also tends to cause more pain problems than anterior instrumentation. Since the back has less tissue to cover the instrumentation, the hardware is often more prominent and thus causes more pain.

Your surgeon, your anesthesiologist, and the rest of the medical staff will do everything possible to minimize the risks associated with surgery, but despite everyone's best efforts, things sometimes happen. Again, every surgical procedure carries with it certain risks, and scoliosis surgery is not exempt from complications. Certainly you should be aware of the risks before undergoing surgery. Yet most of the complications that arise from scoliosis surgery are easily treated and resolved, though they may necessitate a longer hospital stay. Dwelling on risks, focusing all your energy on what might be, will interfere with the positive attitude that can play such an important role in the surgical outcome as well as in recovery.

Revision Surgery

People who have had scoliosis surgery during childhood or early adulthood sometimes develop additional problems related to their scoliosis later in life. Perhaps the bone never completely healed. Or the fusion may have been successful, but curves later developed above or below the area of fusion. Aging, combined with the increased workload placed on discs above and below the fusion, may have caused the discs to degenerate more rapidly, leading to spinal instability and chronic pain. Or the spine may have fused in a malaligned position, typically involving a pronounced flattening of the lumbar spine. When any of these problems develops, patients who have already been operated on for scoliosis may assume that they're stuck. After all, the scoliosis has already been treated, hasn't it?

"My doctor told me that there is help, that I didn't have to just accept what I have. Basically, that's what I was doing," admits Arelene, who suffered from chronic and severe pain owing to malalignment and degeneration. "I had already had surgery, so I thought, 'What else can they do for me?'"

Fortunately, something *can* still be done for you. Further surgical intervention, though often more complicated and less straightforward than your original surgery, can help relieve your back pain and fix what went wrong. An operation performed on patients who have had prior surgery is known as *revision surgery*.

In general, the conditions that may indicate the need for revision surgery fall into one of four categories:

1. *The failure of a previous operation.* By far the most common indication for revision surgery is the failure of a previous operation. A patient may develop a *pseudoarthrosis*, an attempted fusion that never fully heals and fuses, so the area of the spine that should be fixed in position remains mobile. This failure of spinal fusion may result in increasing deformity and/or pain.

2. *The progression of a curve above or below the spinal fusion.* A person may have had a successful fusion performed early in life. But if it was a short fusion, the curve may have progressed above and/or below the fusion with the passage of time.

3. *The development of instability because of disc degeneration above or below the fused area.* Some patients develop problems with instability or disc degeneration above or, more commonly, below the old fusion. A spinal fusion may lead to a need for excessive motion at the levels of the spine that remain mobile. Over time, the discs may wear out, causing instability and back pain.

4. *A fusion that creates a malaligned position.* Some people who have had previous spinal-fusion surgery heal in a malaligned position, so that they are decompensated in one way or another. This poor alignment may result from the poor installation of instrumentation by the first surgeon; decompensation over time, such as the bending of the fusion mass; or some other cause.

"After my first surgery, I felt fantastic. It really relieved the pain," says Susan. "But the Harrington rod broke after eighteen months. They thought at first that it didn't really matter because they say once you're fused, if the rod breaks, you don't need it anyway. But I was losing height, so they knew I wasn't fused. That was very disappointing, because I'd thought it was over with and then it started again."

The simplest type of case to treat with revision surgery involves patients who have a pseudoarthrosis but no malalignment problems. These patients generally do quite well with pseudoarthrosis repair. Through this technique, which greatly resembles spinal-fusion surgery, the surgeon provokes a second fusion, a refusion of at least part of the old fusion. After opening up the back and removing any old hardware from previous instrumentation, the surgeon will roughen up the bone about the area of the failed fusion and add additional bone graft. Often, just one or two areas have failed to fuse properly. So in one sense, this type of revision surgery is less extensive than the original surgery. The surgeon will usually choose to reinstrument the patient, but sometimes a brace worn postoperatively for three to six months will provide sufficient protection while the bone heals.

The group of patients who have had curve progression either above or below the old fusion but remain in good alignment can also expect good results from revision surgery. In these cases, the surgeon simply needs to add on spinal segments to the old fusion. Again, the surgeon will remove the old hardware, install new instrumentation to correct the additional segments involved in the curve, and fuse these segments to the original fusion. In most cases, this surgery can be performed posteriorly. If the additional fusion will extend to the lower lumbar spine, however, the surgeon may need to perform an anterior fusion as well. For example, if the old fusion went down to the L3 vertebra and the extension will go down to the sacrum, the fusion must be performed circumferentially or it will most likely fail.

Many of the patients who develop instability below or above a successful fusion also have some flat-back, or loss of lumbar lordosis, associated with this instability. For this reason, these patients frequently require both anterior and posterior surgery. To correct the flat-back, the surgeon may need to perform one or more *osteotomies*: the surgical fracturing of bone, which involves cutting up a bone, or, in these revision cases, cutting up a fusion. Whereas a fusion results in the creation of a solid piece of bone, an osteotomy begins with either a solid bone or a solid fusion, cuts it into multiple segments, and then re-fuses it in a corrected position. A successful fusion results in a stiff, immobile piece of bone. Yet this fusion essentially fixes the flat-back in place. In order to make it flexible enough to correct, the surgeon will therefore often need to osteotomize the old fusion.

After performing an anterior or a posterior osteotomy—depending on where the previous fusion is—the surgeon corrects the flat-back and then re-fuses the spine. Normal lumbar lordosis, with the convex portion of the sagittal curve at the front of the spine, requires the anterior portion of the lumbar spine to be longer than the posterior portion. In order to correct the flat-back, the surgeon must lengthen the front of the spinal column. To accomplish this, from the front, the surgeon takes out the appropriate discs and puts in "structural grafts"—large grafts, often a solid block of bone that has a mechanical strength to it. Then, from the back, the surgeon corrects the sagittal curve (as well as any lateral curve) and reinstruments the spine.

The most difficult revision cases involve patients who are fused in a malaligned position. This group includes a large number of people who were fused into the lower lumbar spine and instrumented with Harrington rods, leading to a loss of lumbar lordosis, a condition known as "iatrogenic flat-back." (*Iatrogenic* means caused by the physician or medical treatment.) Revision surgery for malaligned patients almost always involves multiple osteotomies and generally requires both front and back surgery. Most patients who have poorly aligned fusions will first need anterior surgery to remove the discs and often to fuse the front of the spine. Then they will also require posterior surgery involving hardware removal, osteotomies, new grafts, and the correction and repositioning of the malalignment through new instrumentation. In these cases revision surgery thus involves more—and technically more complex—surgical procedures to achieve correction than other revision cases do.

Since surgery is often more complicated in revision cases than in original corrective cases, recovery, especially for those who undergo multiple osteotomies and A/P surgery, tends to take longer. Those who have simple re-fusions or fusion extensions also tend to take longer to recover than patients who are undergoing spinal fusion for the first (and hopefully the last) time. But this longer recovery time is not necessarily *due to the surgery* itself. Patients who undergo revision surgery tend to be older, and as age increases, so does the amount of time needed for recovery. Someone who has revision surgery at age 40 will take longer to recover than he did after his first surgery at age 16.

Although perhaps not considered revision surgery in the strictest sense, some scoliosis patients do also need a second operation because of hardware problems. A broken rod, a crosslink, or other hardware—especially in the newer instrumentation systems, which are bulkier than Harrington-rod instrumentation—can be prominent and cause pain in some patients. A bursa, a small fluid-filled sac that may form over the prominent hardware, can become inflamed, redden, swell, and cause intense local pain when touched. Often, this means that patients cannot even sit back in a chair without experiencing pain. If the instrumentation causes this much pain, the hardware, which no longer serves a purpose once the bone has fused, should be surgically removed. Occasionally, a surgeon may be able to avoid a much larger operation by just taking out a small piece of the hardware. If the problem is caused only by the end of the rod or a crosslink, for example, the surgeon might only cut off the end of the rod or take the crosslink off. In many cases, however, pain caused by hardware requires the removal of all of the hardware. This should eliminate the local pain without compromising the fusion itself.

CHAPTER FIVE

Preparing Yourself for Hospitalization and Surgery

"ON AN EMOTIONAL LEVEL, I WAS REALLY VERY CON-cerned about the operation," says Susannah, recalling the months leading up to her surgery. "I don't know if I blew it out of proportion in terms of my fear, but I was very intimidated. It was difficult because I felt that I really was all alone in certain respects. Of course my parents were incredibly supportive, and my friends were sweet and supportive, too. But there was really no one I knew who was going through what I was going through. It wasn't like the feeling of a big history test with thirty kids all having that same anxiety. I really was the only one.

"During those few months I got frustrated very, very easily. I just got fed up with my thirteen-year-old friends' little problems and quibbles about life. It was a weird time. It was hard for me because I'd go to school and I'd be like a normal kid and I'd be dealing with people who were worrying about homework and tests and I was thinking of how after school I'd have to meet with my parents and some doctors and X-rays and just be terrified."

Like Susannah, you or your child may find the weeks or months between the time when you decide to have surgery and the time you actually enter the hospital an intense and anxiety-ridden period. After all, you will be undergoing major surgery that will change not only your posture, but your body image and perhaps the quality of your life. Though you may welcome these changes as ends, the means of achieving those ends, the process of change, can be intimidating.

"I thought something would be changed somehow," Susannah continues. "I thought that somehow I would be different physically from the operation in such a big way that I could never return to how I was before. Or emotionally different. And because of that, in the months beforehand I felt like I was readying for some kind of big change. It sounds weird, but I remember I made a photo album of my life, I wrote a lot of short stories and poems. It was a very introspective time."

Any kind of surgery brings with it a host of legitimate fears and concerns as well as general anxiety. And spinal surgery obviously carries more anxiety with it than, say, leg surgery. As Karin notes, "It is an unbelievably frightening experience, the idea of someone splitting open your back." Despite your doctor's reassurances, you may fear complications, the effects of anesthesia, paralysis, even death. The fact that the risk of serious complications is very low may have little impact on your fears. Fears may have a rational basis (the concrete *possibility*, however remote, that these things could happen), but they do not always respond to rational arguments (a realistic assessment of the *probability* that they will).

Finding out as much as you can about the operation, hospitalization, and recuperation may ease some of your anxieties, though it may not cause your fears to disappear entirely. Start by asking your doctor any and all questions you might have. You will likely have many of the following questions that my patients have asked me:

- What does the surgery feel like?
- Is it painful?
- How long will the surgery take?
- How much correction can you hope to achieve?
- How serious is this operation?
- Could I die from this operation?
- Could I end up paralyzed?
- What will I be like after I wake up from surgery?
- Will I look different or feel different afterwards?
- How long will I be in the hospital?
- When will I be able to walk, bathe, enjoy sex, drive?
- How much school or work will I have to miss?
- What are the kids or adults who have had this surgery like now?
- Will I be able to have a normal life and have children and play sports and do all those physical things?

You probably have other questions relating to your individual situation. Don't worry about whether you are asking the right questions or intelligent questions or appropriate questions. You have the right to know everything that will happen in the operating room and during the rest of your stay in the hospital, and how it will affect your life.

"Ask questions," Arlene urges, "because I think it does help, if you're going to go into surgery, to know what's expected, to know the pain that you're going to have. I just wanted to know the ins and outs. I know that helped me tremendously to come out of the surgery fine, to progress out of the intensive-care unit, and to get on to the floor and to get myself up. That's the type of person I am."

Since this period is difficult for most patients, I usually schedule several appointments—at least two and sometimes more—prior to surgery and encourage patients to call if they have any questions they forgot to ask me during these meetings. You might find it helpful to write down your questions as they occur to you so that you will remember them in the doctor's office. During these office visits, I try to tell my patients everything about the procedure they will be undergoing. I want them to know very specifically what to expect in terms of the surgery, the hospital stay, and recovery at home. I'll talk about pre-donating blood, about the different parts of the surgery, about the aftercare, about the expected activity level after surgery. Yet try as I might, I cannot anticipate all of a patient's questions and concerns. That's why you need to ask questions: to get your doctor to address *your* specific concerns.

Many of my surgical patients find it very helpful to talk to other patients who have had similar surgery. As Susannah notes, no one else really knows what you're going through. Your doctor may be sympathetic, your family and friends may be incredibly supportive, but unless they have had the surgery themselves, they cannot tell you what it really feels like from the patient's perspective. For instance, I try very hard not to underestimate the pain and illness associated with procedures performed to treat scoliosis. But there's really no way I can tell a patient how much pain he will be in after surgery, so I offer every patient the option of talking to other patients who have had similar surgery. Although some people never avail themselves of that opportunity, those who do almost always find it helpful.

"I thought it would be depressing to talk with kids who had the surgery," recalls Susannah. "And I kind of thought, 'Oh, I don't need it.' I was in denial in a way. But about five nights before my operation, I was in bed and trying to go to sleep and for the first time it really dawned on me that apart from all the emotional, weird, abstract, general ideas I had about it, in five days I would literally be in a hospital having an operation. It would be me, it wouldn't be this weird fictional me I had been worrying about.

"I went in and I told my parents and I just started crying and I said, 'There's nothing you can do about it. I'm not going to *not* have this operation, but there's nothing you can do to make me feel completely at ease about the fact that this will happen.' When I went to school the next day, I tried to find comfort in my best friends, and they were comforting, but they *really* didn't know how I felt.

"Then finally, the night before I was supposed to go into the hospital, I called a girl who lived in New Jersey and we talked for about six hours. And I said, 'Is it painful?' She said, 'It's not so much painful as it is just uncomfortable. I don't know how to explain it but you'll know exactly what I mean when it happens.' She was right."

As Susannah and many other patients have discovered, no one understands the flood of feelings and fears that can overwhelm a person facing scoliosis surgery better than someone who has already gone through the experience. You or your child may feel that the upcoming surgery sets you apart from your family and friends. No doubt you have special concerns, pre-surgical worries, profound fears, and intense feelings that your doctor, your friends, and your family cannot share, despite their caring. The experience of having been there before lends your fellow scoliosis patients an authority that even your doctor and your family cannot have in this matter.

In addition, people who have already undergone scoliosis surgery can often serve as a reliable source of hope and promise. They can offer detailed, real-life stories of how the operation changed their lives—stories that carry much more emotional weight than any information your surgeon can relate. "People who call really want to know how well I'm doing now," says Rachel, who has informally counseled several of my patients since her own surgery. "They like hearing that I had a forty-degree curve and now it's about six or seven degrees, that I've never had one instance of recurring backache and pain since completing my recovery, that when I put my clothes on, my pants are totally straight and I no longer have to hem my skirts slightly crooked."

If the informal counsel provided by your family, your doctor, your friends, and any former surgical patients fails to ease your most profound fears and feelings, you may want to consider seeking professional counseling prior to surgery. After surgery, Betty suffered from a number of medical complications includ-ing pneumonia, an allergic reaction to the anesthesia, and a painful ileus that led to postsurgical feelings of depression. She wishes in retrospect that she had received some professional counseling prior to surgery. "The doctors do prepare you for the possibility that things may go wrong," Betty acknowledges, "but you just assume they're just listing things, especially when they start with, 'Well, the worst case would be you could die.' I think that patients should have counseling of some type before they go in for surgery, because if I had been a little more calm and relaxed and prepared for something to go wrong, I would have done better."

You should probably talk to someone, whether your doctor, your friends and family, or a psychologist or other professional counselor. That's why I always give my surgical patients the names and telephone numbers of others who have had the same operation in the past. In describing what she tells those who call her for support, Susannah provides insight into why it can be so valuable to patients facing major surgery for scoliosis: "First of all, I say that the fact that you're talking to me is really good, because it's important not to feel alone. I also say to tell your parents and your friends that you are afraid, and it's not just a piece of cake, and don't just brush it off because that'll just come back to haunt you later. And third, I don't know if I can guarantee it but I say that things will work out. And that if you are brave and you just get through this, that within a matter of months, you will be able to go back to your old life, but it will be better because you won't have to worry about it all the time. I say that it's going to be better than you think."

Planning for Surgery and Aftercare

Any hospitalization and surgery requires a certain degree of planning. Scoliosis surgery, which typically involves a one- to two-week stay in the hospital and six weeks to six months of recovery, demands a great deal. In the weeks prior to surgery, you will need to attend to a number of details that will help your hospitalization, surgery, and recovery proceed smoothly. Some of these details center on logistics—setting a date for surgery, making sure someone will help take care of you when you return home, settling insurance questions, etc. Others involve medical concerns—a physical exam, X-rays, pre-donating blood, etc. The final details focus on preparing for hospital admission—pre-admission tests, consent forms, packing, fasting, etc. Here's what you'll need to do, in roughly this order.

1. Setting a Date

In the weeks following surgery, you will have little energy to devote to your personal, work, or school life. You won't want any loose ends or obligations hanging over your head while you're trying to concentrate on recovery. Susannah took this into account in deciding on the timing of her surgery. "Eighth grade was an incredibly important year," she explains, "in terms of my friends and teachers and family, because I knew it would never be like that again, that intimate middle-school feeling. I didn't want to be 'the girl who missed school to have an operation.' I wanted my spring break, too, and I wanted to graduate from middle school in style and spend time with my friends and family and not have to worry about it. And summer seemed like the perfect time. I got to have a real rejuvenation in privacy. I got to take my time. I think if I had been in school, it would have been very difficult dealing with missing work and being worried about catching up and having to go back to school and get stares from people about why I haven't been there for so long. I think that would have added a whole new level of difficulty."

In choosing a date for your surgery, remember that you are

not dealing with a medical emergency. Unless you are experiencing severe pain, a few months more or less will make little difference. Even a rapidly progressing curve in a young adolescent will only grow 6 to 8 degrees in six months. So schedule the surgery at your convenience. Certainly, a minimum of six weeks of recovery time is never convenient, but consider when the best time would be for you and your family.

2. INSURANCE

Whether you personally can afford it or not, you can always find surgical care available through one source or another. If you have a standard health insurance policy, after meeting your deductible, you should be covered for 80 percent of the cost of scoliosis surgery. If you belong to an HMO, the cost of the operation may be covered in full, although your HMO may not allow you access to the specific surgeon you want. Virtually all insurers today cover scoliosis surgery. I would advise contacting your insurer as soon as possible after making the decision to go ahead with surgery. This will give you time to obtain a letter of medical necessity—which confirms that it's not merely cosmetic surgery—though very few insurance plans require a second opinion to testify to the medical necessity of the operation.

If you are uninsured, you may have to absorb the cost of scoliosis surgery, which varies greatly from region to region. If you have no insurance and no means to pay for surgery, you can still receive good surgical treatment through clinics like the one in our hospital, the Hospital for Joint Diseases Orthopaedic Institute, in New York City. You can also receive free surgical care for your scoliosis if you are on Medicaid. In addition, Shriners

Hospitals will provide free care for children in need up to the age of 18 or 21, depending upon the individual hospital. So if you live near a Shriners Hospital, you may want to contact them to discuss treatment.

3. Setting Up Aftercare

Many people tend to focus on preparing for the hospitalization itself, but you should also plan ahead for your return home, when you will likely be in no shape to do much of anything for yourself. If you have parents or a spouse or friends living with you who will care for you, you may not need to worry as much about how well you will function when you get home. But especially if you live alone, you'll need to make adequate preparations for your at-home recovery. Stock up your freezer with easy-to-prepare foods. Arrange for friends or relatives to drop in and check on you at regular intervals when you get home. Obtain home and work numbers for those willing to assist you and put them next to the phone. If you think you have special needs or circumstances—for example, if you live alone in a fourth-floor walk-up—let your doctor know. The doctor's office can sometimes involve social-service agencies to ensure that you receive adequate care when you return home or to arrange for a physical therapist, if needed, to come into your home after surgery.

4. X-rays

You will need to provide a full set of current X-rays prior to surgery. Standard preoperative X-rays include:

- a standing anteroposterior (A-P) or posteroanterior (P-A) X-ray, preferably on a long plate to give a full view of the entire spine from the base of the skull down to the sacrum;
- a standing lateral X-ray, also preferably on a long plate; and
- left and right supine bending X-rays.

In addition, especially if the patient has neuromuscular or degenerative scoliosis, the orthopedist may request:

- forced bending X-rays;
- traction X-rays; and/or
- push-and-pull X-rays.

X-rays provide the best information on a scoliosis patient's condition before surgery so the surgeon can assess what can reasonably be expected from surgery. Most important, X-rays serve as an indispensable tool for surgical planning, for example, to determine what the limits of the fusion need to be.

Since your doctor will make surgical decisions based on your X-rays, you will need to provide current ones. Any X-rays taken less than three months prior to surgery will serve this purpose unless you or your child has grown rapidly in the interim. So if a good A-P X-ray was obtained six weeks earlier as part of the decision-making process, your doctor may not ask you to replace it with a new one. Even though it is not always necessary to do so, however, some surgeons like to obtain a full preoperative set of X-rays, including an updated A-P film, just to make sure the surgical team has a full set of films prior to surgery. If your most recent standing A-P X-ray was taken more than three months prior to the operation, you should definitely get a new one.

The procedures for getting A-P, P-A, and lateral X-rays were described in Chapter 2. To obtain a bending X-ray, the radiologist will ask you to lie down supine (on your back), put your right arm over your head, and bend as far as you can to the left. After the machine, poised above you, takes an X-ray of you in this position, the radiologist will ask you to switch, putting your left arm over your head and bending as far as you can to the right. Another A-P X-ray will be taken in this position. Taking these two X-rays while you lie supine eliminates the effect of gravity, thereby giving your surgeon some idea of the flexibility of the curve. Bending your back laterally provides the surgeon with even more information about the potential for correction. For instance, if a standing X-ray shows a 50-degree curve and a supine right bending X-ray shows a 20-degree curve, the doctor will know that the curve is so flexible that simply by bending, the patient achieves a correction of 60 percent. Surgery should therefore be able to do at least that well. In addition, bending X-rays help your doctor decide exactly how long the fusion needs to be—whether to include all the curves or just do, for example, a selective thoracic fusion.

People who have idiopathic scoliosis do not generally need to get "forced benders," traction films, or push-and-pull films to help in presurgical planning. They are reserved primarily for cases involving neuromuscular or degenerative scolioses, which may prevent patients from bending on their own or giving their best effort. To obtain a forced bender, an X-ray technician wearing a lead apron and lead gloves manually bends you as you lie in a supine position. To obtain a traction film, you lie supine on the table while someone grabs hold of your head and someone else your legs. The X-ray is taken as they both pull. A push-and-pull film requires you to lie prone, on your stomach, so that your rotational deformity, or rib hump, is up. By applying pressure to the deformity, and therefore to the apex of the curve, the radiologist or technician can obtain an X-ray that offers more infor-

mation on sagittal curves than the standard lateral X-ray. As
pressure is applied to the rib hump, someone else can pull on the
patient, as in traction films, to lengthen the spine. These techniques provide a better estimate of the flexibility of the curve or
curves, the potential to correct them surgically, and the potential
for correction of any sagittal deformities secondary to scoliosis.
They can also help the surgeon assess which surgical approach
would be most appropriate: posterior, anterior, or both.

5. PRE-DONATING BLOOD AND THE ALTERNATIVES

I would strongly recommend that all patients who are able to
pre-donate their own blood (called "autologous" blood donation) do so as an outpatient in the weeks prior to surgery, so that
it can later be used for transfusion during surgery. The safest
blood for you to receive through transfusions is your own blood.
By donating your own blood, you avoid the need to put anyone
else's blood in your body. Transfusions of your own blood eliminate the risk, however small, of acquiring AIDS or other infec-
tious diseases, as well as the risk of an incompatibility reaction.
I can't think of a patient who, given today's risks, would not
want to donate his or her own blood. Unless you have anemia,
there's really no good reason not to do it.

Even young children can pre-donate their own blood. Although children who weigh less than 75 pounds should probably not donate a full unit at a single time, blood banks do not
always need to take a full unit of blood. Children can donate a
half unit, even a quarter unit, at a time. Some blood banks are
unwilling to take less than a full unit, because the amount of anti-
coagulant in the standard bags in which they collect the blood is

calculated on a full unit of blood. This means that the blood bank will have to prepare special bags for children who donate less than a full unit, but there's really no reason they shouldn't do this. If you need to donate less than a full unit of blood, contact your blood bank to find out whether they will accommodate you by preparing a smaller bag in advance.

The amount of blood needed for your operation will depend upon the nature of the procedure. I typically ask my patients to donate two units of blood for a routine anterior or posterior procedure. If the patient needs a longer fusion and the operation will therefore involve greater blood loss, I may ask for three or four units. If the patient will be undergoing complicated front and back surgery, I ask for six units of blood. Donated blood lasts for 35 to 42 days, and you should *not* donate any blood during the week of surgery. So if you need six units for complicated surgery, you will need to begin donating a unit per week five or six weeks prior to surgery. If more is needed, you can begin donating earlier and freeze the blood.

If for any reason you cannot or will not pre-donate blood for autologous transfusions, alternatives do exist. You can arrange for donor-directed blood, meaning you pick the person, a family member or friend, who donates the blood. Although this is not quite as safe as using one's own blood, parents of younger children sometimes find it preferable to donate their blood for their children's surgery.

Other techniques can come into play in the operating room to minimize your need for a transfusion in the absence of pre-donation or directed donation. The surgical team should use an intraoperative cell-saver, which salvages blood used during surgery and immediately retransfuses it into the patient.

The surgical team may also use a very effective technique

called hemodilution, or auto-transfusion. As soon as you are brought into the operating room and put under anesthesia, the team removes one or two units of your blood and replaces it with a plasma expander or volume expander—usually isotonic saline, Ringer's lactate, or albumin. This dilutes your blood (making you acutely anemic during the surgery), so that during the operation, you lose only diluted blood. After the operation has been completed, or before, if necessary, the whole blood, which has been stored in a refrigerator, can be retransfused into you.

Another alternative that can minimize your need for nonautologous transfusion involves manipulating the blood count by administering prior to surgery erythropoietin (EPO), a hormone first developed for treating chronic anemia in patients with kidney failure. EPO stimulates the marrow to produce more blood cells, giving patients "supernormal" hemoglobin counts of 16 or 17 rather than the normal hemoglobin level of 13. With high hemoglobin counts, you can afford to lose more blood. Although this works very well, it is very expensive, about $1,500 for one course of treatment, and many insurance plans won't cover it. So if you want this technique employed for your surgery, you'll probably have to pay for it out of your own pocket.

Finally, the surgical team can do a postsurgical transfusion, which involves catching and salvaging the drainage of blood that has accumulated after surgery. During your operation, blood drained from the wound is collected in a reservoir. Instead of throwing this blood out, which was standard practice until recently, the surgical team can put it through a special filter and then retransfuse that processed blood through your intravenous tube. While the intraoperative cell-saver elaborately washes and cleans the blood before retransfusing it into the patient, postsurgical transfusion merely runs it through a filter to remove gross impurities. Thus this technique involves putting back unwashed though filtered blood, which may have collected particulate debris, and may cause medical complications after surgery. Consequently I avoid using this technique unless I regard it as absolutely necessary.

Although all of these techniques have demonstrated their effectiveness in reducing patients' need for nonautologous blood transfusions, the safest, most effective, and least expensive alternative is pre-donation. So even if giving blood tends to make you queasy or faint, I still urge you to do so. If you do choose to pre-donate blood, your doctor will probably ask you to take iron pills to help build up the blood during the period of your donations.

6. PHYSICAL EXAMINATIONS

Whether or not you need a physical exam prior to surgery depends upon your specific medical condition and history. I generally ask all children and teenagers to have a brief exam done by their pediatrician a few weeks before surgery. I also generally require patients over the age of 45 to have a routine physical. In addition, if someone has a history of a medical problem, I'll often have that person cleared by the appropriate internist or specialist about a week prior to surgery. For example, if a child has a history of congenital heart disease, I make sure I've seen an up-to-date cardiology report and perhaps an echocardiogram prior to surgery. Most patients, however, who have no particular medical history, do not need any special medical exam prior to surgery.

7. CONDITIONING AND FITNESS

If the patient is a normally active teenager or younger child, there's probably no need for any special conditioning program prior to surgery. But I encourage all adults and less active children who are preparing for surgery to go on an aerobic fitness program prior to their hospitalization. "One thing that was helpful in recovering from the surgery was getting in good physical shape beforehand," Karin says. "I was very conscientious about that. Just being physically strong was helpful in other ways, too, because after surgery you have to use other muscles to pick things up when you can't bend over." A typical aerobic fitness program consists of brisk walking, using a treadmill, riding an exercise bike, or swimming for at least 30 minutes every other day. If you have adopted a sedentary lifestyle, this simple aerobic fitness program may seem a little difficult at first, but it doesn't really place any rigorous demands on you. If you want to pursue an even more aggressive and active course of exercise and fitness, I would encourage you to do so. In general, the stronger and more fit you are prior to surgery, the quicker and easier you will find it to recover afterward.

I don't usually regard weight as an issue prior to surgery. A patient's nutritional status has a much greater impact on recovery than her weight. Poor nutrition can interfere with an individual's ability to heal. If a patient is very thin, I might check her nutritional status. A teenager who has anorexia will tend to be nutritionally deprived. In such cases I try to get the patient in good nutritional balance by the time of surgery.

8. PREADMISSION TESTS

About a week prior to your operation, hospitals require a bat-
tery of preadmission tests in order to admit you for surgery.
Generally, these consist of routine blood studies, urinalysis, X-
rays (if necessary), and a preadmission physical examination.
This includes a general physical exam (heart, lungs, abdomen)
as well as an orthopedic exam (description of deformity, etc.).
Adult patients who have reached a certain age, which varies
from state to state, may also need to have a rectal examination
(men), a pelvic examination (women), a cardiogram, and/or a
chest X-ray.

Preadmission tests are usually administered at the hospital
four to seven days prior to admission. This time frame allows all
blood work to remain current upon admission, but allows time
for all results to be in prior to admission, providing an opportunity to evaluate and check any abnormal results. A recent preadmission test for a 15-year-old girl showed that she had a
minor blood-clotting abnormality. As soon as I got the results, I
sent her to a hematologist, who thoroughly evaluated the condition, determined it was not serious, and okayed her for surgery
as scheduled.

During your visit for preadmission tests, you should also
meet with your anesthesiologist. The anesthesiologist performs
an evaluation and asks whether you have ever had any problems
such as nausea or allergic reactions with anesthesia during any
previous surgery. This also gives the anesthesiologist an opportunity to explain the type of anesthesia she plans to use, to tell
you what you will likely experience in the operating room, and
to answer any questions you may have regarding possible risks
and complications.

If you have the time, I would suggest using the preadmission tests as an opportunity to familiarize yourself with the hospital. If you will be undergoing an anterior procedure, arrange to see the intensive-care unit, because after surgery you will remain in this unit until the chest tube is removed. Children in particular find it helpful to see the hospital and become familiar with the environment, but I believe that most adults find it beneficial, too.

9. PACKING

You really don't need to bring much to the hospital. For the first few days after surgery you'll be provided with a hospital gown. Though you can wear these gowns throughout your stay, most people feel more comfortable in their own clothing after the first few days. So you might want to bring a nightgown or a pair of pajamas and a comfortable bathrobe; avoid clothing that needs to be pulled over your head. Remember to bring slippers for walking around once you're back on your feet. Socks are also a good item to have to ward off any chill. Bring toilet articles such as toothbrush, toothpaste, hairbrush, comb. The hospital can no doubt provide you with all of these, but they will seldom be as nice as your own. You may want to bring a book or a magazine, but most people find that the postoperative painkillers make it next to impossible to concentrate on much of anything. *Don't* bring much money; you won't need more than a few dollars, for a TV hook-up, for example, and you will have no way to safeguard your money.

10. HYGIENE

We ask patients to shower thoroughly prior to surgery to make sure they're clean. You don't need to use any special soap for presurgical scrub. If you have long hair, it would be helpful to braid it prior to admission to keep it out of the way during surgery. Scoliosis surgery seldom necessitates shaving any body hair. Even for anterior procedures, it's probably not necessary to shave any pubic hair unless the operation will go very low down on the spine. If pubic hair does need to be shaved, you don't need to do this yourself.

Especially if you will be undergoing an anterior procedure, the hospital or your surgeon may ask you to have an enema prior to surgery. Most scoliosis patients are not admitted to the hospital until the morning of surgery, so you may need to do your own enema at home. Those hospitals and surgeons who require presurgical enemas do so for two reasons. First, since a clean bowel reduces the risk of infection, the enema purges the bowel, just in case it is nicked during surgery. Second, the sphincter, like other muscles, relaxes when people are put to sleep, and an enema can help prevent soiling the operating table. If this happens, the whole O.R. will need to be broken down and cleaned up. I have seldom seen this happen, though. For this reason, I almost never require enemas anymore for any surgery, although we used to do them routinely, and some surgeons still do.

11. FASTING

Since food in the stomach increases the risks associated with anesthesiology, especially the risk of regurgitating and choking on the vomit, you should not eat or drink *anything* after midnight the night before surgery. If you have had as little as half a glass of water within eight hours of surgery, anesthesia should not be administered. This eight-hour fast will allow your stomach to empty itself completely prior to surgery.

12. INFORMED CONSENT

Either before admission or upon admission, you must sign two informed-consent forms. In the first form, you agree to allow the hospital to treat you. It does not refer to any specific surgical treatment, but rather allows you to be treated within the institution. The second form gives your specific, informed consent to undergo scoliosis surgery. The discussions you've had in your doctor's office prior to surgery provide the basis for this informed consent. Once you sign it, you've agreed to allow the doctor to perform the operation. Now you're ready for surgery.

CHAPTER SIX

What to Expect in the Hospital

"THE NIGHT BEFORE SURGERY, A NURSE ON THE floor interviewed me," recalls Alison. "And I said to her, 'How many people when they're going down the morning of the surgery burst out crying and become hysterical?' And she said to me, 'Lots of people cry.' But then she said to me, and we laughed about this all the time afterward, 'But Barney says it's okay to cry.' And just having laughed about that sort of made everything all right."

The hospital can be a frightening place, especially if you're facing major surgery. But it may help ease some of your fears to know exactly what will happen once you get there. As a surgeon, I can describe the various procedures, the surgical instrumentation, the monitors used, and other precautions taken to increase the safety of the operation. But having never had scoliosis surgery, I cannot personally offer you a sense of what the experience is like for a patient: the colors, the emotions, the flavor of what will happen to you. For that, I depend upon patients like Alison and Susannah, Karin and Rachel, Arlene and Betty and Susan. Their voices of experience will tell you what it feels like.

"We went in the afternoon of the day before," Susannah remembers. "That night was kind of like the calm before the storm. People were being overly nice to me and a little delicate and handling me with kid gloves. I wasn't even afraid because it was so near. It was like there's nothing I can do. Nothing can be said or done at this point to change anything, so I might as well wait for time to pass. I just felt at peace with things."

Although, like Alison and Susannah, patients are sometimes admitted the day before surgery, if you are scheduled for posterior or anterior surgery, you will typically be admitted to the hospital on the morning of surgery, probably around six A.M. In either case, you should have had nothing to eat or drink since midnight the night before surgery. A member of the nursing staff and a medically trained member of the house staff—a physician, a physician's assistant, or a nurse practitioner—will admit you. A nurse will perform a nursing assessment, asking you a list of precautionary questions such as: Do you have dentures? Do you know what your operation will be? How many units of blood have you pre-donated? If you did not have a history and physical taken as part of preadmission procedures, someone from the medical staff will do these upon admission.

After admission on the morning of surgery, you will be prepared for the operating room. You will be asked to undress and put on a hospital gown. "They woke me up at five o'clock in the morning, maybe even earlier, to prep me for surgery," Susannah recalls. "And I specifically remember two nurses braiding my hair in pigtails to keep the hair off my back during surgery. And the nurse gave me a shot in my arm which made me very woozy."

After these preparations have been completed, the transportation staff will put you on a gurney and take you to the operating room fully awake and conscious. "I remember being very calm when I went down in the morning," says Alison. "I guess when you're at that point it's very impersonal. Like the person who takes you down, he's not necessarily going to talk to you and hold your hand and be nice to you. His job is simply transportation." Susannah also recalls the transfer to the operating room as a calm time: "I remember them coming in with a stretcher-type thing and my getting on it and just feeling so relaxed with the whole thing. I remember waving good-bye to my parents and them telling me everything would be all right, they'd see me when I woke up. I remember being taken to an area which was clearly right outside the operating room and waiting there for a long time."

In the Operating Room

In the operating room you will see tables piled high with surgical instruments. For many patients this can be an intimidating and even overwhelming sight. "I thought it would be dark and womblike," admits Alison. "It's not. Bright and loud and people doing their thing all around you. They come, they put you on the table, and they strap your feet in, which I didn't know. Then you realize this is really happening. That was surprising. Everybody's talking about everything, chatting away. I feel like I'm the least important person there. And I'm thinking, 'Hey, this is my big day.'" The operating room will be filled with people bustling about, doing their jobs, talking to one another, and hopefully trying to help you feel at ease. The operating-room staff generally consists of a two-person anesthesia team (an anesthesiologist and often a nurse anesthetist); one or more scrub nurses, who will be scrubbed and will assist with the operation; one or more circulating nurses, who will be responsible for getting the equipment the surgeon needs; the surgeon; and an assistant surgeon—a resident, fellow, surgical colleague, or physician's assistant—who will assist the primary surgeon throughout the operation.

"I met my anesthesiologist," remembers Susannah, "and he shook my hand and said, 'Hello, Susannah, I'll be your anesthesiologist today.' He was joking, the way someone would say, 'Hi, I'm Steve, I'll be your waiter tonight.' And then he said, 'I want you to count from ten backwards.' It was just like in the movies. And he put the I.V. in my hand and I looked down and I saw a vein in my hand rise and I counted down from ten to nine to eight. And then at about eight there was this swirl of colors and the room started swirling. Again, it sounds like in a movie, but I really did feel like images of my life and my family were all kind of swirling into this big red and green image in my head, and that was it."

Typically, scoliosis surgery itself takes about three to four hours, although large curves in adults generally take longer. You will spend much more time than that in the operating room, however. The anesthesiologist first needs to put you to sleep, the O.R. staff needs to position you correctly on the table, and following surgery, you need to be awakened. These procedures add perhaps one or two more hours to the time you spend in the operating room. If you are scheduled for an 8:00 A.M. surgery, you will be brought into the operating room around 7:15. The initial incision will be made at about 8:30 and the operation will be finished at around 12:30. By the time you are taken out of the operating room, it will probably be after 1:00 P.M.

While you remain awake, the only procedure that will be performed is the insertion of an intravenous line, generally into a vein in the arm. This I.V. will be used to administer anesthesia, retransfuse blood, and provide fluids as well as perhaps some sugar. It will also supply antibiotics, administered for 24 to 48 hours to prevent infection. After the anesthesia has been started through the I.V., you will probably remember nothing else until you arrive in the recovery room. Everything else that happens in the operating room will occur after you have gone under anesthesia.

Once you are anesthetized, a Foley catheter will be inserted to drain urine out of the bladder and an endotracheal tube will be passed down into your throat and hooked up to a respirator. The endotracheal tube will allow the anesthesiologist to safely control your breathing during surgery. Most patients have no memory of the endotracheal tube, since it is generally removed just as the patient is waking up. Occasionally, however, with a very long operation, the endotracheal tube might be left in the throat until the patient is fully awake, responsive, and breathing comfortably on his own. The anesthesiologist wants to make sure that the patient is fully awake and safe before disconnecting the respirator. Since the need to leave in the endotracheal tube typically occurs in patients who have longer procedures, it can generally be anticipated and forewarned. For example, if you are undergoing major surgery from both front and back, your surgeon or anesthesiologist will warn you that you may still have the endotracheal tube in when you wake up.

The anesthesiology team will then hook you up to a variety of anesthetic safeguards. A cardiac monitor allows the anesthesiologist to keep track of the functioning of your heart. A pulse oxymeter, a device that fits over one finger, provides a continuous reading of the oxygen saturation of your blood. An arterial line, a blood line in an artery in the wrist, constantly monitors your pulse and blood pressure. Since the surgical team will lower your blood pressure with drugs in order to reduce bleeding during surgery, the blood pressure must be monitored very carefully. A spinal-cord monitoring technician or the anesthesiologist will also attach appropriate electrodes for spinal-cord monitoring. The spinal-cord monitor provides a continuous reading of spinal function and thus provides surgeons with the earliest possible warning of any damage to the spinal cord. Since the spinal-cord monitor is removed at the end of the operation, you will not wake up with these electrodes attached.

Finally, the surgical staff will put pneumatic compression boots on your legs. These boots are attached to a machine that sequentially blows them up and relaxes them, simulating the effects of muscles contracting, which keeps blood pumping through your veins. This significantly reduces the risk of blood-clotting diseases such as thrombophlebitis, an inflammation and clotting of the veins, typically in the legs. Although thrombophlebitis itself is not a big problem, it creates the danger that a clot will break off and go to the chest, causing a pulmonary embolism, a potentially fatal disease. To guard against this complication, these pumps remain on your legs after surgery until you are fully ambulatory.

For a typical posterior procedure you will be positioned facedown on the operating table after the surgical staff has fully prepared you for surgery. Different kinds of operating tables are available; I use a Jackson table, which supports the patient throughout the chest and the pelvic areas, but reduces blood loss during surgery by allowing the abdomen to be free, thereby eliminating much of the pressure on the blood vessels that drain blood from around the spine. Once you have been positioned, your back will be scrubbed for 10 minutes with an antibacterial scrub solution. The surgical team will drape most of your body, so that all they can see is the patch of skin on your back through which the incision will be made. After making the incision, your doctor will perform the surgery, as detailed in Chapter 4.

Typical anterior surgery involves the same preparatory steps as posterior surgery: You are hooked up to a Foley catheter and I.V. line, intubated by the anesthesiologist, and connected to the various monitors that guard your safety throughout the operation. In addition, in anterior surgery a nasal-gastric tube is inserted through one nostril, which decompresses your abdomen, removing gas and fluid so that the belly remains flat and not distended. This is necessary because anterior surgery can interfere with normal peristalsis, the contractions that push intestinal contents forward. The nasal-gastric tube prevents the accumulation of gas and fluids in the intestines that could cause distension, discomfort, and vomiting for 24 to 48 hours after surgery.

You will be positioned on your side, with the side to which the curve bends facing up. This is the side where the incision will be made. If you have a left lumbar curve, you will be positioned on your right side so that your left side faces the surgeon. After scrubbing and draping you, the surgical team will make the incision and perform the surgical procedure.

After finishing the surgical procedure, but before closing you up, your surgeon may perform a *wake-up test* to satisfy herself that no neurological damage has been done. The surgeon asks the anesthesiologist to reduce the anesthesia to such a level that you wake up. Since drugs will be used to paralyze you temporarily during the surgery, so that the spinal-cord monitor will work properly and the surgical team can do their work in a motionless field, the surgical team must first make sure that these drugs are no longer in effect before performing a wake-up test. After bringing you up from the anesthesia, you will be asked to wiggle your toes in order to evaluate the status of motor function following the insertion of the corrective hardware. Although it sounds gruesome to wake someone up before closing up the surgical wound, the test causes no pain in any way and patients almost never remember it. Nonetheless, patients should know prior to surgery that it might happen.

Wake-up tests, which for many years served as a standard of care for scoliosis surgery, are performed less and less since the advent of good spinal-cord monitoring. Some surgeons still wake up every patient after the hardware is inserted, because they regard spinal-cord monitors as not reliable enough to reflect all damage that may occur. Although this is perfectly reasonable and appropriate, I no longer routinely use wake-up tests. I feel comfortable relying on today's state-of-the-art spinal-cord monitors, which provide a continuous reading of both the sensory and the motor part of the spinal cord, whereas the wake-up test assesses gross motor functioning only for one particular moment. I use a wake-up test only if a technical problem with the spinal-cord monitor crops up during the procedure, if the spinal-cord monitoring looks abnormal, or if I have any concern that some damage might have been done to the spinal cord.

After your doctor closes the incision using a dissolvable stitch, a dressing is applied. An X-ray is generally taken to doc-

ument that all hardware is in place. You will be transferred from
the operating table onto the gurney or stretcher, and moved
to the recovery room, also called the postanesthesia care unit, or
PACU. You will remain in this unit for one or two hours until
you are fully awake.

"It felt like there was no time lapse at all," Karin recalls. "I
remember being sort of groggy as I was heading toward surgery.
My husband was with me and after a point I think he wasn't allowed to go any further. And then, it seemed like the next
minute, the doctor was saying, 'Karin, it's over. Wiggle your
feet.' It felt like there was no time lapse.

"Then I was in intensive care. I was pretty out of it. The
biggest memory of that is just trying to clear my throat. But I
wasn't in awful pain."

When you wake up in the recovery room, you will still be
hooked up to a lot of I.V. lines and machines. A suction drainage
tube in the incision will remove the blood that accumulates after
surgery, thereby helping to prevent hematomas, accumulations
of blood clots under the skin that increase the risk of infection.
If you have a thoracoplasty, you will have a second suction drain
tube at this site. In addition to the I.V. line supplying fluids, nu-
trients, and antibiotics, you will now be hooked up to a patient-
controlled analgesic, or PCA, an I.V. line attached to a morphine
pump for the administration of pain medication. The pneumatic
compression boots will continue to keep blood flowing through
your leg veins, and the Foley catheter will remain in place to
drain urine from the bladder. The pulse oxymeter and the leads
for cardiograms, if removed following surgery, will be put back
on in the recovery room to allow continuous monitoring of your
cardiac functioning, blood pressure, and the amount of oxygen
in your blood. If you have undergone a long operation, you may

still have an endotracheal tube in place until the anesthesiologist is satisfied that you are breathing well enough. If you've had an anterior procedure, a nasal-gastric tube will exit through one nostril and a chest tube will exit your chest from a separate incision on the same side as your surgical incision. Its purpose is to help prevent a collapsed lung by equalizing pressure in and draining fluid from the chest cavity.

"When I was in the recovery room, I was in pain," Susannah admits. "It was no fun being there. But I really couldn't care less because I was so thrilled to have this weight off my shoulders that I had been worrying about for years. It was incredible."

A Little Better Every Day: Hospitalization and Recovery

"You wake up and you can't move," says Karin, who had eight vertebrae instrumented and fused. "You can't even roll over by yourself. You can't do anything by yourself initially. But what was very encouraging was that every day you can do something more. And every day it gets a little better."

Most patients who undergo surgery for scoliosis remain in the hospital for about a week after surgery, or about 10 days for those who have had both anterior and posterior surgery. Following your stay in the recovery room, you will be moved to a regular hospital room. (If you have a chest tube because you've had an anterior procedure, you will go to the hospital's intensive-care unit for three to four days.) Ideally, the hospital should have a step-down unit, a mini-ICU where patients would go from the recovery room for the first day or two after surgery, and also a floor where all scoliosis patients go for the remainder of their stay. But most hospitals, including ours, do not have the facilities to operate this kind of unit. At our hospital, we have one floor where most spine patients go.

Most people wake up from surgery feeling unable to do much of anything. "I was at everybody's mercy," says Betty, who had an anterior discectomy and fusion as well as posterior osteotomies and instrumentation to reposition a previous fusion. "I couldn't do anything myself. I couldn't get out of bed, couldn't roll over in the bed, couldn't get into the bathroom by myself, couldn't even reach over and get a bedpan." Although complete bed rest is not mandated on the day after surgery, don't expect to do much except lie around. You won't be asked to sit up or get out of bed or do much of anything. Certainly, if you want to get up to go to the bathroom and feel comfortable doing it, go ahead. But most patients don't want to do anything on this first day.

"What happens is you have your surgery, and you're basically almost a mummy," Rachel explains. "You're kind of wrapped up, you can't move, you have all these bandages, you have tubes sticking out of you." Although you probably won't do anything, things will be done to you. The hospital staff will reposition you every two hours or so, "logrolling" you from your side to your back and then again to your side. This helps prevent bedsores, which can form if you remain in one position for too long.

You won't feel very good. You may feel short of breath. You will feel exhausted from the anesthesia and the surgery itself and groggy from both the lingering effects of anesthesia and the narcotics used to deaden the pain. Despite these painkillers, you may still feel achy.

"One thing they didn't warn me about that was frustrating was that I couldn't drink fluids for two days afterwards," Susannah complains. "Obviously, I had an I.V., but I couldn't drink and so I was incredibly thirsty. People had to come and wipe my mouth with damp washcloths."

Most people have little desire to eat after surgery. Though you may feel very thirsty, as Susannah did, you will be much better off going very slowly with eating and drinking. Many patients develop a postoperative ileus, a failure of the intestines to contract normally. If you eat or drink too soon after surgery, the ileus will cause your large bowel to become distended and you may vomit. To avoid this possibility, you will be given neither food nor drink on the day after surgery.

Your overall view of your hospitalization will depend on many factors: the promptness and quality of care provided, your own personality, and any complications that might arise. Alison says, "The hospital experience is awful. You fear that if you call somebody, they're not going to come. And that's worrisome, at least it was to me. I remember I couldn't wait to get out. I think that as soon as you get home, you're better off. You will be cared for by your loved ones, and your level of anxiety goes down."

Rachel, who had a rib removed for bone graft and four vertebrae instrumented and fused, agrees with Alison. "I had a terrible time at the hospital," she admits. "That's definitely the worst part of the experience for me. In retrospect, my family and I would have done it very differently. I realize now that in a hospital situation, you really need to be the squeaky wheel, and if you're incapable of doing that, your primary caretaker, whether that be a husband, mother, father, or whoever, has to be unafraid to ask questions, to be persistent and just make sure the staff is aware of what your medication is, what you're getting, why the nurse is taking twenty minutes to clean a bedpan, things like that."

A hospital can be a very frustrating place. Since nurses have to take care of an entire floor of patients, they have to balance your needs and desires with those of all the other patients on the floor. Your doctor may be seeing patients all over the hospital, too, making it difficult for him to give you the intense attention you may feel you need. The entire hospital staff will do their best to keep you feeling as comfortable as possible, but they cannot constantly be available to any one patient. And this can be very aggravating, especially during the first day or two after surgery, when you will be totally dependent on others to do *anything*. "If you can afford it," Rachel suggests, "I would definitely recommend hiring a private nurse for the first forty-eight hours after surgery if your hospital doesn't allow a loved one to stay with you twenty-four hours a day."

Though some patients find the hospital frustrating, their own dependence irritating, and the hospital staff incredibly slow and unresponsive, others view the hospital as the best possible place in which to recover from surgery. "It was really nice," Susannah says. "I was just thrilled to be done with my operation. The nurses were incredibly sweet. It was a great time. I just felt so free and happy for the first time in a very long time. I watched TV, I read books, I wrote letters to my friends, I got tons of phone calls and letters from my friends, and flowers. It was great. I loved it.

"Sure, there were things that weren't so great. I had to roll over all the time to prevent getting bedsores and I was just generally sore. Having a catheter in for the first day or two afterwards was really unpleasant. Sometimes I felt kind of gross because I hadn't showered in a while. I just felt as if everything was moving in slow motion. Usually my life is so busy, riding the crosstown bus, going to school, doing assignments, and talking on the telephone. The pace in the hospital was just very slow. I remember the feeling of having all these flowers in the room, this kind of very heavy, sweet air, and things moving very slowly."

The Course of Postoperative Pain

"They tell you you're going to be in pain," Alison acknowledges. "And I know that you can't tell a person what pain is like. I had been told that I had a very high threshold in relation to pain, so I thought I'd be able to manage it. But it was extraordinary how difficult it was to move afterwards. You can't even lift your head up. It was like being an infant again."

Surgery for scoliosis is a big operation and therefore a painful one. The pain comes at you from many directions. You may feel pain in your back, in your legs, in your belly, and in your side. "My biggest complaint after the surgery was the muscle pain," says Arlene, who had both anterior surgery and posterior surgery. "That was hard. I would be sitting and all of a sudden the tears would just come out. I would literally cry, but it was just the tightening of all the muscles. I had such pain down my left side, all the way down my leg, and in the left buttock, that I couldn't even walk five feet without crying. I have none of that now, though, no pain at all."

While in the hospital, you can expect pain from the incision, pain at the site where the graft was taken, and pain throughout your whole back. Any postoperative ileus will tend to cause stomach pain as well. Since it will also hurt around the back of the hip, you may find yourself limping, dragging the leg on the side from which the graft was taken, for a few days after surgery.

"Some of the most extreme pains aren't even at all directly related to the back," warns Rachel. "I didn't feel any pain in my back for a long time. Of course, most of the pain is concentrated where they removed bone for the graft, so in my case it was my ribs. But I also had terrible gas pains, which no one warned me about. The pains also cause a tremendous surge in your body temperature, not necessarily fever, but you get cold sweats and chills, and they're very uncomfortable and scary if you don't know what's going on."

Curiously enough, as Rachel notes, some scoliosis patients don't feel any back pain for some time after surgery. Also, the more intense pains that come from the site of the bone graft or from the distension of the intestinal tract often overshadow back pain in the initial postoperative period. Some patients even contend that "pain" is not quite the right word for the feeling they have in their back.

"It felt very tight in my back," Susannah explains. "It felt like there was metal tape all down my body, which was from so much bandaging. It felt very taut. It was a weird feeling, having some metal thing attached to my back somehow.

"So for the first two days after my operation, there was intense discomfort. I just wanted to crawl out of my skin. I felt weird and kind of tight and I could sense strange things going on in my back. But I guess after the second day, when I got up and I started walking around, things got easier. It was so wonderful, and I got exponentially better every single day so that by the third day I was completely walking around, by the fourth day I had no tubes and I was eating and going to the bathroom on my own. By the fifth day I felt like a person recuperating from any other illness. So the discomfort was not that prolonged."

Before you have surgery, it's very important that you understand how the pain can be expected to progress. Most people expect the most intense pain to occur immediately following surgery, then gradually and steadily to diminish over the next few weeks. But because of the effects of anesthesia and narcotics, the most intense pain generally occurs one or two days after surgery. Furthermore, postsurgical pain does not follow a steady course, decreasing bit by bit until it disappears completely. Rather, it involves a lot of ups and downs, with these fluctuations coming rapidly in the first few days after surgery. I draw for my patients a graph of the pain they can expect to experience after surgery, which looks something like this:

INTENSITY OF PAIN

DAYS AFTER SURGERY

You may feel great one day, so you get out of bed and do a lot more walking, maybe try some stairs, and exert yourself a great deal. The next day, you may feel so awful that it's a struggle merely to sit up in bed, much less get out of bed and walk around as much as your doctor, physical therapist, and nurse insist. The resurgence of pain may become frustrating and disheartening. But if you anticipate these vacillations of pain and recognize them only as temporary setbacks, however stressful they may be, they will not cause you to lose hope in your recovery.

"I actually thought the pain was going to be much worse," says Susan, who had revision surgery involving both anterior and posterior fusions, the removal of old hardware, and the insertion of new instrumentation. "And I was really surprised it wasn't that horrible. My hospital uses those new morphine pumps now, so that really helped, I think."

The intensity of pain following surgery demands treatment through narcotic pain medications. For the first two to three days after surgery, you will be hooked up to a patient-controlled analgesic. The PCA gives you a degree of control over how much pain medication you are taking. It provides a basal rate, or minimum, of narcotic every hour, and in addition to this you can give yourself additional medication as needed up to a predetermined maximum per hour. Some people do have a problem managing their own medication. Perhaps fearing an overdose or because of excessive stoicism, they tend to undermedicate themselves and therefore bear unnecessary pain. *You cannot overmedicate yourself with a PCA* because the computer is programmed to prevent this. You could click the button a thousand times in an hour and the PCA will still only give you the maximum amount safely prescribed and programmed into the machine. Over the course of two or three days, the amount of morphine provided will be titrated, or gradually decreased, to wean you from it.

"I was on a morphine pump. That made everything much easier," Susannah says, "because psychologically I felt in control of my pain. And I couldn't give myself too much because there was a limit programmed into it. That was immensely helpful. And because I couldn't feel the pain so much, I really was able to walk around and do all the stuff I wouldn't have been able to without the morphine."

Susannah was just 13 years old when she had her spinal fusion, and she too felt pain and needed narcotic pain medication. It's very important that both parents and hospital staff avoid *under*medicating children. Though children tend to recover more quickly than adults, they feel postoperative pain, too, and they will recover more quickly and comfortably if this pain is managed appropriately. Children do not need as much pain medication as adults. The actual narcotic dosage is calculated according to the surface area of the child's body, and this adjusted dosage will be programmed into your child's PCA.

Like any medication, narcotic painkillers can cause side effects or adverse reactions. Virtually all narcotics tend to cause some constipation, light-headedness, and weakness. Less common but nonetheless possible reactions to analgesics include nausea, sweating, rash, and/or transient hallucinations. Karin experienced some respiratory depression on morphine. "There was a sensation during the night one time when I felt I was having trouble breathing in kind of an indescribable way," she says. "I was told after the fact that morphine slows down your breathing or it can give you this feeling. I was much happier on Percocet than morphine."

Rachel developed a highly allergic reaction to the morphine she received postoperatively: "My fever went up to a hundred and four, I developed a rash and started swelling all over my body," she says. "And they had to take me off all the painkillers and put me on Demerol right away, which is usually given four or five days after surgery. Usually, they give you morphine for the first three days, because it's the strongest painkiller. And then you take the next strongest for three days. And Demerol is the third strongest. But with my allergic reaction, they put me on that right away. So within three days after my surgery, I was already down to Tylenol with codeine. So unfortunately, I got stuck with all the weak painkillers. And the codeine tends to cause constipation, which worsens the gas pains."

Constipation is common in the aftermath of scoliosis surgery. Indeed, virtually everyone gets constipated following surgery—especially anterior surgery, which necessarily involves at least some manipulation of abdominal contents. When smooth muscle such as that in your digestive tract is manipulated, it becomes "lazy" for a while. This laziness can lead to the development of an ileus, a paralytic distension of the intestines. Narcotics, which reduce the motility of both the bowel and the bladder, tend to exacerbate both a postoperative ileus and constipation. For this reason, I tell all of my patients that even if they use laxatives, stool softeners, or suppositories, their bowels will not function normally and regularly again until they're home and off most narcotics. Iron supplements can also cause constipation. Most patients begin taking oral iron supplements when they start to pre-donate blood and continue taking them until the day before surgery to mitigate postsurgical anemia. Since the combination of surgery, narcotics, and iron can cause severe constipation, you may need to discontinue taking iron supplements until you've been weaned from your pain medication.

Do You Need a Postsurgical Brace?

Most scoliosis procedures performed today, whether posterior or anterior, do not require the patient to wear a postsurgical brace or cast. Postoperative braces can help preserve and protect the instrumentation and area of fusion until the bone has healed. However, the segmental instrumentation systems used today are so much stronger than the systems once used that bracing has become unnecessary in most cases. Nevertheless, I still do brace approximately 5 percent of my surgical patients. Most commonly, I brace older patients whose bones have become softer. In such cases, concern about the quality of the fixation of the instrumentation into the bone suggests the need for a postoperative brace. This decision is based entirely on the surgeon's experience, knowledge of bone, and judgment. If the surgery has been undertaken to correct a very severe deformity, this might also warrant the use of a postoperative brace. Finally, I might consider postoperative bracing for patients who undergo complicated revision surgeries. Since these operations involve a lot of hard work for both doctor and patient — surgery from front and back, 12 hours in the operating room, plus previous surgery — I almost routinely brace these patients after surgery just to avoid the need to bring them back into the O.R.

Postsurgical braces are usually custom-made TLSOs (thoracic lumbar sacral orthoses), low-profile underarm braces. These plastic braces provide an external shell to support the internal fixation. A postoperative brace must be fitted after surgery because your shape will have changed. Sometimes orthopedic surgeons can make a mold of the patient right on the table in the operating room and the brace maker can manufacture the brace during the first few days after surgery, while the patient is still in bed most of the time.

If you are reasonably thin and the surgery achieved good correction, you may be measured for a stock (prefabricated) brace a day or two after surgery and the orthotist will make the brace from these measurements within a few days. If you still have significant, persistent deformity after surgery, you may have to wait a little longer because the orthotist will have to make a custom brace. To make a mold for the custom brace, you lie on a special table and the orthotist applies plaster to form a "jacket." She waits until it hardens, and then takes off the plaster jacket and makes a mold of your body from it. It takes four to five days after surgery before a patient can lie comfortably on the molding table, and then it takes several more days to make the custom brace. For this reason, a person who needs a customized postoperative brace must stay in the hospital slightly longer than others.

Typically, if you need to wear a brace, you will wear it only for upright activities. This means you need not wear it to bed, you can take it off to shower, etc. The horror stories of scoliosis patients who spend a year or more after surgery in a back brace or cast are rarely seen today. Instead, most patients who do need postoperative braces typically wear them for just four to five months.

"The brace itself is made out of fiberglass now, so it wasn't cumbersome at all," says Arlene. "I didn't care if I had to wear it or not, I knew that this was going to help me and I knew I had no choice. As for mobility in the brace, I had no problem with that either, because I wanted to do what the surgeon had told me to do. Just trying to bend, to put my shoes on, was a challenge, but I think it was because of the surgery itself."

Patients who need braces after surgery tend to tolerate them more readily than adolescents who need to wear them until they achieve skeletal maturity. Postoperative braces have a significant advantage in that the time for which they will be needed is always limited, ranging from three to six months, whereas an adolescent needs to wear a brace for an open-ended period — two years to five years or more, depending on when bracing begins. In addition, unlike adolescents who wear braces to prevent curve progression, patients who have gone through surgery gladly accept a brace because they want to preserve the correction the surgeon has achieved. Finally, many patients feel more comfortable in their postoperative braces than they do out of them. The external support provided by the brace reduces the stress and strain on the muscles, which are already sore and irritated from the surgery.

"I wore a brace for about four months after surgery," says Alison. "Once it was fitted, I didn't find it to be difficult at all. I found it actually harder to take the brace off. When I went for my first checkup, about five weeks after surgery, I had to go for an X-ray. The technician said, 'You have to take the brace off for this X-ray.' And my first reaction was 'I'm not allowed to take it off.' Eventually I had to take it off, and it felt awful. I had a tremendous anxiety attack and didn't know why. That week, I had a nightmare; I dreamed I was falling. And I woke up and immediately realized that it was the same experience I had when I took the brace off. That feeling lasted for quite a while. Even when I first started taking the brace off for an hour at a time, I'd still have that sensation."

After you've been wearing a postoperative brace regularly, your muscles will often feel sore and achy when you take off the brace because they have to do more work when the brace is not supporting them. So you may go through a period after removing the brace in which you feel an increase in discomfort and pain. Some patients have described this sensation as feeling as if the back will collapse. Despite this sensation, your back will not actually collapse. Appropriate physical therapy can usually resolve any increased discomfort, pain, or feeling of imminent collapse.

Getting Back on Your Feet

Although you won't feel like moving a muscle on the first day after surgery, you will be up and about as soon as the pain starts to diminish, generally within two or three days. Granted, you probably won't have the usual spring in your step. At first, even the simplest tasks will present a challenge: sitting up and putting yourself in an erect position, getting in and out of bed, getting to and from the bathroom, getting on and off the toilet seat, walking to a chair across the room. All of these will tend to cause pain and exhaustion during the first days after surgery.

By the second day after surgery, a nurse will have instructed you on how to use an *inspirometer*, a device that exercises the lungs. It connects a breathing tube to several columns, each of which contains a ball. Blowing into the tube, causing the balls to rise in their columns, exercises the lungs, expanding the alveoli (the lungs' air-containment cells) and preventing them from collapsing, which could easily lead to a pneumonia. I usually tell my surgical patients to breathe into it for 10 minutes every hour that they're awake. Even this may initially seem exhausting.

Patients who undergo posterior surgical procedures typically begin drinking within about two days of surgery. So you may start to sip a little water by the second day. Those who undergo anterior surgery are more likely to have a postoperative ileus and will still have a nasal-gastric tube in place for one or two days after surgery, so they will progress more slowly toward drinking and eating. Once the abdominal muscles and organs begin to work more normally again, you won't need the nasal-gastric tube and can begin to progress toward a normal diet over the course of several days, beginning with clear fluids, then a soft diet, and a normal diet by the time you leave the hospital.

On the second day you may perhaps sit up in bed a little bit, for up to half an hour at a time. You may even dangle your legs over the side of the bed, but the trauma of surgery will make even this difficult. You can expect wooziness, fatigue, achiness, and soreness.

By the second or third day, you may stand at the side of your bed for a short time. And by the third or fourth day, you will probably begin walking, with the assistance of a walker for a day or so if necessary. "After the third day, I was up walking around, which was a big deal," says Susannah. "The first day I walked my physical therapist took me down some stairs and back up some stairs. I remember they were *much* more difficult even than the walking was. But the more I walked and the more I was active, the better I felt."

Like Susannah, most patients view these first small steps as a giant leap in their recovery, but walking too will not be easy. Pain around the hip area on the side from which the graft was taken may cause you to drag the leg on that side. This type of postoperative limp, very common among patients who've had scoliosis surgery, should not be a cause for alarm. In addition, if you have had an anterior procedure that involved the removal of discs, you may find that you pitch forward a little, that your balance feels a little off. Yet despite these difficulties, most patients find that walking makes them feel immediately better and speeds recovery in general.

"It's quite a surprise when they have you get out of bed the next day and walk," Karin admits. "The feeling I had after surgery wasn't excruciating pain, I was just very sore and stiff. And I would walk around the hospital corridors in the middle of the night just because it would feel good to move the limbs and make me feel less sore and stiff. So I would take a little tour with the nurse."

By the fourth or fifth day after surgery, you will probably have achieved a certain degree of independence. You may be able to get out of bed on your own, to walk independently, and to get to the bathroom without assistance. You may even be able to take a shower. Physical therapists, occupational therapists, and nurses will provide training in all these daily activities and others, such as getting up and down stairs, getting dressed and undressed, and getting back into bed. Before you can be safely discharged from the hospital, you will need to know how to do all of these activities on your own.

Most of the tubes, I.V.s, and other attachments that kept you safe, managed your pain, and substituted for normal body functions in the first few days after surgery will be disconnected by this time, adding to the growing feeling of independence. The drainage tube from your incision will have been removed around the second or third day. If you are drinking enough, the I.V. will be removed by the fourth day, as will the catheter if you can get to the bathroom on your own. Around this time, you will also discontinue use of the PCA and instead take narcotic pain medication orally, as needed. If you have difficulty controlling your pain, the medical staff will evaluate you and possibly put you on a pain program. This may consist of round-the-clock administration of pain medication by the nursing staff rather than having it available on request. The amount of medication given to you will be gradually decreased prior to discharge.

Most people stay in the hospital for five to seven days after surgery, or a few days longer if they have had both anterior and posterior surgery. Prior to your discharge, a staff physical therapist will evaluate your need for any specialized tools at home. If needed, the hospital can provide a toilet-seat extender, a walker, a cane, or any other tools you might need. On the final day of hospitalization, an erect X-ray will be taken to document the degree of correction achieved by surgery. This X-ray will provide a base line, allowing the orthopedist to compare follow-up X-rays to make sure that you haven't lost any correction or developed other problems.

A New You

"For some reason I thought that the first time I saw my scar would be a very difficult, scary, depressing moment and that I would remember it forever," Susannah says. "I was terrified of the first time that I was going to take off the bandages and see it. But when I took them off, it really looked fine, and I was surprised at that. I actually have grown to love my scar, I'm proud of it. I've never tried to wear things that cover it up."

By the time you leave the hospital, you will most likely be able to walk without any assistance from either people or devices. Although you still won't feel great, you will feel much better than you did immediately after surgery. You will have a low tolerance for sitting, walking, and exercise, but you will certainly be able to do all of these things, most of them on your own. And you will feel and look physically transformed.

"I felt kind of like a new person because I had become taller from the operation, about three inches taller," Susannah adds, feeling justifiably proud of herself. "I literally woke up and I was taller. It was incredible because I walked around when I first stood up and it felt like wearing high heels. Things were this much taller, I mean higher, I mean lower," she says with a laugh. "That was incredible. And my body was different because it used to be kind of crooked and now it was straight, perfectly straight, which made me just feel so happy about myself and my body and my confidence."

Like Susannah, you will gain height through corrective surgery for scoliosis. If you had discs removed, this will decrease some of your height gain, but the correction of the curve will add even more height than the discectomies lose. Most patients gain anywhere between ¾ of an inch to two inches, depending upon the size of the curve prior to surgery. In addition, you will feel more balanced when you stand or walk. Finally, your rib hump will generally be smaller, particularly if you have undergone thoracoplasty. These physical changes can have an enormous impact on how you feel about yourself.

"It was just an unbelievable feeling afterward," Karin confides. "This has been basically hanging over my head for twenty-five years. It's quite a feeling to be done with all that. And so I've said to different women who've called me and seem to be anticipating the worst that they should just have the operation. No pun intended, but just put it behind you. It's a really good feeling to have it over with."

CHAPTER SEVEN

Recovering from Scoliosis Surgery

ALMOST EVERYONE WHO HAS HAD SURGERY TO COR-
rect scoliosis ultimately views it as a positive experience. Even
during the most difficult periods, the first days in the hospital
after surgery and the first weeks at home after discharge from
the hospital, you will have something positive and tangible that
can sustain you in your efforts to recover. Just look at yourself
in the mirror. You will see that you are straighter and taller.
This new appearance, as Susannah noted, can give you a confidence boost that will help accelerate your recovery. For most
people, the physical transformation that results from surgery
makes all the hardships of recovery not merely bearable, but
worthwhile.

"I liked the immediacy of it," Rachel explains. "The first time
I got out of bed and looked at myself in the mirror, I immediately
saw the difference in my body. I took pictures the day before
surgery and about a week after surgery, and you could see a

tremendous difference just in the hip level. So I consider myself a raging success story. The quality of my life has improved tremendously. Actually, sometimes I think that this is the best thing that could have happened to me, that I was lucky it happened when I was still young. It's great that it happened the way that it did."

Feelings of relief, confidence, and gratitude are not uncommon responses to scoliosis surgery. Even when operations don't yield results as dramatic as those in Rachel's case—her curve was reduced from 40 to 7 degrees—patients still tend to feel different about themselves, better about themselves, after surgery. And these feelings of renewal can carry them through the challenges of recovery. Karin's curve was reduced from 67 to 25 degrees. "It looks basically straight to the eye at this point," she says. "But I still have sort of a hump on one side. He couldn't get rid of that totally, where my ribs have been sort of squooshed to one side. And I have one shoulder blade that's noticeably a lot bigger than the other. But he did straighten my back a lot and so it has made a big difference.

"I can wear clothes I never wore before. I had trouble before wearing suit jackets because they wouldn't lie smoothly on me. But now I can wear more form-fitting and tailored suit jackets. Actually, where I still have a little bit of a hump, a tailor does sometimes put a little pad in the back on the other side, just to even it out. Also, before surgery, if I put a belt around my waist it would be higher on one side than the other. My hips were way off. Now that's not a problem. And that's an encouraging thing for a woman: that if you're going to go through all this awfulness, at least you'll look better, too."

Going Home: An Emotional Journey

Usually before I perform surgery, I try to let patients know what will be expected of them as they recover from surgery. I don't want *anything* to come as a surprise. This guiding philosophy applies to every detail about surgery and recovery: procedures, the amount of correction, complications, the degree of pain, challenges, the duration of recovery. I believe that everything you experience during surgery, hospitalization, and recovery should be something that you've at least heard about before, something familiar to you. If a patient and her family members are adequately informed beforehand, it will be much easier for them to face the significant challenges of the postoperative period. I think that a large part of the doctor's job after surgery involves setting targets for patients: establishing goals and letting them know approximately where they should be in the process of recovery. This goal-setting, coupled with positive reinforcement, helps get patients through the demanding and sometimes frightening process of recovery.

Surgery is scary. Understandably, you may have a lot of fear after surgery. You may, for example, fear that if you stand up at all or walk or fall down, you're going to fall apart. And the pain that will come as you engage in these activities will only strengthen your sense of panic. The fact that the instrumentation in your back is solid and reliable may have little impact on this profound fear. Knowing how much surgery has transformed you, you will be hesitant to do anything that might risk destroying all that work.

"You feel very, very fragile and vulnerable," Karin says. "You go for a walk and you're always looking behind you. You go into a restaurant and you want to sit with your back against the wall so nobody can bump you. I just wouldn't put myself in crowds where I could get bumped. The first time I went into New York City, I had to really watch my way. I felt very vulnerable back there, though the fear lessened over time. But it's quite a feeling."

As Karin indicates, your sense of vulnerability will probably dissipate as time passes and your healing progresses. However, this feeling may never go away entirely. Especially during the first six months, before the bone has completely fused, you will feel particularly insecure. Having just been through surgery, you will know what an ordeal it can be and you will likely fear the possibility that you might have to undergo surgery again. You will want to do everything you can to protect your surgery. Unfortunately, the back is perhaps the most unprotected part of your body.

"I remember I felt incredibly vulnerable for a good four or five months afterwards because the back is one part of your body you can't see," Susannah explains. "I found myself looking behind my shoulder a lot. Even in school the next year, people would come up and give me a good, hearty slap on the back, and not only would it hurt, but it would also freak me out because I would feel like there's so much harm that could be done to me and I would have no idea."

Many of my patients have expressed this sense of vulnerability in the wake of surgery. I explain to them that the instrumentation itself provides a great deal of protection for the healing spine. That's the reason it's there: to hold the healing spine in place no matter what your everyday activities may be. If your surgeon has any reason—soft bone, for instance—to be concerned about possible dislodgement, he will put you in a postoperative back brace to provide further protection. Despite this reassurance, the fear may remain.

Some patients have little fear for their backs, but feel vulnerable about other areas involved in the surgery. In particular, the site of the bone graft, perhaps because it tends to cause even more pain than the back itself, can feel unprotected and susceptible to outside dangers.

"I still tend to protect my left side in the area of my ribcage, where a rib was taken out and where my scar is," says Rachel. "I can feel a missing rib when I run my hand over my ribcage, an indentation where the rib was and no longer is. I feel very protective of that area. If my husband is turning over at night, the first thing I do is just naturally kind of cover that spot with my hands." You too may feel an instinctive need to protect your back or your ribs following scoliosis surgery.

In addition to a heightened sense of vulnerability, surgery can also sometimes lead to a flood of other fears. Some of these—a fear of heights, hypochondria, or claustrophobia—may seem indirectly related to scoliosis, or to your desire to protect the corrective surgery and to avoid further hospitalization. But others may seem entirely unrelated to the scoliosis surgery.

"For about a year after my operation, I had lots of little fears," Susannah says. "I had been very brave about the operation beforehand and I really didn't ever tell anybody what I was feeling. I think I needed to wait to release it. I became afraid of flying in a very intense way. So I think definitely my fear of the operation presented itself by spreading out."

To help deal with your postoperative fears and other feelings, you may want to seek some professional counseling. It may also help to talk to other surgical patients who are further along in recovery than you are. "Everybody's experience is a little dif-

ferent, but I found it really helpful to talk to other patients,"
Karin acknowledges. "And when I felt better, I wanted to recip-
rocate." Just as they can help ease fears and answer doubts
prior to scoliosis surgery, your fellow scoliosis sufferers can
offer comfort, reassurance, and motivation in the months after
surgery, too. For this reason, in follow-up visits with current patients I frequently offer the names and telephone numbers of
former patients who have had similar surgical procedures. Not
everyone takes advantage of this opportunity, but those who do
generally find it helpful. Jill felt miserable about six or seven
weeks after undergoing complicated front and back surgery for
scoliosis. She felt a lot of pain and doubted whether she would
ever get better. I put her in touch with Mary, who had undergone similar surgery a year earlier. When Mary told her that she
had felt miserable for three to four months following her
surgery, it quieted some of Jill's doubts and fears. She still felt a
lot of pain and knew that she would continue to do so for a couple of more months. But now Jill knew that this was normal and
that she could reasonably look forward to a time when she
would not feel so much pain.

In addition to talking to peers and/or professionals, continue
to consult your orthopedist regarding your doubts, concerns,
and fears. I ask my patients to call if they have *any* questions or
problems after they go home. In most cases, people who call do
so because the area around the wound has begun to swell or
they feel more pain than they think they should or they wonder
if they can drive a car yet. Most patients only want a little reassurance that what they're going through is normal, or practical
guidance about how much they need to restrict their activities.
Your doctor can readily supply this guidance and reassurance,
so don't hesitate to ask if you want or need help.

The counseling offered by your orthopedist, a professional psychologist, or your fellow scoliosis patients can also provide you with comfort, understanding, and advice during those times when you feel postoperative depression or frustration. Recovery can be an extremely frustrating process. Just as the course of pain following surgery features highs and lows, so the course of postoperative emotion fluctuates. One day, you may feel completely better: pain-free, active, and ready to take on any challenge. The next day, you may feel terrible: exhausted, unable to move without pain, miserable.

"Four weeks after my surgery I went back to the doctor for my first postsurgical checkup and X-ray," Rachel recalls. "I remember that was a severe day. I was not in pain, but I was terribly exhausted and very depressed because I still didn't feel at all great. You're worried about this before surgery, that it's going to take a while to feel good, but you kind of feel like that applies to other people, that you'll be fine. I really thought after two weeks I'd be on my feet again. So to find myself after a month still not feeling great, still in a lot of pain, was really depressing."

Temporary setbacks may understandably leave you feeling depressed, anxious, impatient, and/or frustrated. Particularly if you had a pain problem prior to surgery and you still have pain after surgery, you may succumb to the depressing notion that you'll "never get better." Despite the fact that you will in time feel better, you may quite reasonably lose faith in the course of recovery when pain recurs.

Emotions do not adhere strictly to the rule of reason. Your frustration or depression may have a logical cause, but it may also come "out of nowhere." Postoperative depression may result from repression of these feelings prior to surgery—as Susannah suspects. Repressing these emotions may have been necessary to get you through the operation, but they may come back in a flood at an unexpected time after surgery.

"It's true about the postoperative blues," Rachel says. "There was a week when I did nothing but weep. It was about six weeks after my surgery when I finally felt pretty okay. I was still in bed most of the day but feeling much better. And all of a sudden, there were three or four days when the smallest thing could make me weep all day long."

Recovery from major surgery leaves one feeling both physically and emotionally vulnerable. You will need not only physical support when you return home, but also emotional support. Recuperation invokes not only elation, triumph, giddiness, and pride, but also intense fears, anxiety, depression, doubts, loneliness, and vulnerability. Since these emotions can interfere with the physical work you will need to do in order to advance recovery, they demand attention. So make sure you have someone—a close friend or relative, another scoliosis surgery patient, a professional counselor, or your doctor—with whom you can share these feelings. Asking for the support you need will help speed your recovery.

Returning to the Activities of Daily Living

"People were sending me books to read, thinking that this is time off, that I was on my back," Rachel remembers. "And I am a big reader, but I had absolutely no ability to concentrate in that state. I lived with the remote control in one hand, and that's all I did. I would doze off most of the day. Even a TV movie called for too much concentration. So I lived on a diet of Jenny Jones and Oprah for three weeks straight. I had thought, 'Oh my God, I'm going to have two months off from work. This is great. I'll just relax.' But it wasn't like that. You need the two months just to concentrate on recuperating."

When patients are discharged from the hospital, I tell them that they can do almost anything they feel comfortable doing at home. I encourage patients to set their own limits, rather than looking to me to tell them what they can and cannot do. Even though I do not restrict postsurgical activities, I recognize that the process of healing will initially impose severe limitations on what most people can do. Children generally recover from major surgery very quickly, perhaps within a month or six weeks. But most adults don't have the same resilience and adults generally feel more pain. In general, the older the patient, the longer it will take to recover fully from major surgery and return to the activities of daily living.

"When I got home, my doctor told me I could do whatever I wanted, because I think he knew I couldn't do anything," Susan says with a laugh. "I mean, absolutely nothing. Even if I had wanted to do something, it was physically impossible. I would say I didn't feel great for at least six weeks. But that's to be expected. And then as I felt better, I started doing things. I think by six weeks I was pretty well on the road back to normal."

I encourage patients to get back to their normal level of activity as quickly as they possibly can. But this will take time. In addition to pain, the primary factor that limits postsurgical activity is sheer exhaustion. "You're extremely tired," says Alison, "that's the amazing thing, how tired you are. I remember that I wanted to walk, not only because walking supposedly helps the fusion, but I thought if I was walking, I was surviving. So when I came home, what I would do is walk a little bit, then go back to bed. I was exhausted."

Postoperative fatigue stems from many sources. Surgery it-self is traumatic, causing the body to focus most of its energy on healing and leaving little energy for much of anything else. In addition, the time spent in bed causes a certain degree of atro-phy in the muscles, which become "lazy" from disuse. Trying to use these muscles again as you recuperate thus generates not just soreness, achiness, and discomfort, but also fatigue. Finally, the after-effects of anesthesia, which may remain in the system for one to two weeks after surgery, also tend to produce exhaus-tion.

"Even taking a shower was an event. I got tired very, very quickly," Karin recalls. "Everything was a challenge. I was ex-hausted and felt like I was going to be exhausted the rest of my life, but that's not true. The anesthesia makes you very tired for about ten days. Once that leaves your body, you're naturally less tired. And then everything got to be less and less strenuous."

In deciding what you can and cannot do upon returning home, it's very important to listen to your body, to pay attention to your body's pain and fatigue reactions as you undertake cer-tain tasks. Your body will tell you what and how much activity you can tolerate. This does not necessarily mean that you should stop what you're doing at the first sign of pain or fatigue. Con-tinue to challenge yourself, pushing yourself to get better. But don't push yourself too hard or try to do too much too fast. Your body will send signals that will help you decide how much is too much.

"I got back home and mentally I felt I could handle anything because I had already been through this and I really had noth-ing else to worry about. Everything else just paled by comparison," Susannah relates. "So I felt I could do anything. I remember my first meal when I came back from the hospital. I was so hungry that we went to McDonald's because I hadn't had bad-for-me food for a while. But afterwards I was sick because I had eaten nothing but hospital food for a long time. I had to lie down and I realized that there was a lot my body was not able to do that my mind felt I should be able to. My mother and I would take walks around the block, and even a week and a half to two weeks after my operation, it was difficult. I'd come home winded after a block."

I instruct patients going home after surgery to be as active as they can be *comfortably*. It's important that you not stay in bed all day, because staying in any one position for too long may increase your stiffness. At first you may need assistance to get in and out of bed, but you will be doing it on your own within the first week. For the first day or two, just walking across the room to sit in a chair for a half hour or so may seem like plenty of activity. Simply sitting up may cause additional pain and may also bring on wooziness or dizziness. Yet the more you do it, the easier it will get. You may find it more comfortable if you have some pillows in the chair—for example, a small one to place behind the lumbar spine. Even then, you may find it difficult to find a chair that seems comfortable during the first week or two after getting home. To avoid additional stiffness, try not to stay in any one position for too long. Don't just plop down in a chair for four hours in front of the TV. Change position in the chair often, and after 30 or 45 minutes, get up again, walk around, do some stretching. Try to be active.

By the time you return home, you should be able to go to the bathroom by yourself. The most difficult part of using the toilet is sitting down and getting up. You may therefore find it helpful to spend twenty dollars for a toilet-seat extender, so that you don't have to sit down as low on the toilet. You can probably buy one at the hospital or a local medical supply company.

You can probably shower on your own, within a week or so of returning home, but you might need help drying off, since bending and reaching back will be challenging and painful. Even if you don't need help in the shower or afterward, you might find it comforting to know that someone is down the hall or outside the bathroom door in case you do need something.

You will need more help during this initial period at home than at any other time in your recovery. For this reason, says Karin, "I actually brought a private-duty nurse home with me for a shift just to show me how to show someone how to help me do stuff at home. And then I had somebody helping me for two weeks. And then my son's nanny was here helping me after that."

If you have young children, you will also need help. Although you can hold a baby and do many aspects of child care, you will find it next to impossible to lean down into a crib and pick up a baby, at least at first.

Patients with small children often wonder whether they should avoid lifting the baby—or anything else heavy. I generally tell patients that they can lift up to 25 pounds in the first few months after surgery. Whether you are picking up a toddler or a box of books, you must first know how to lift correctly. Always bend your hips and knees rather than bending at the waist, and always face what you're lifting, instead of trying to twist around and lift at the same time.

To build muscle strength and prevent stiffness, take short walks—maybe for the first few days only to and from the bathroom or to and from a chair, but soon up and down stairs and then outside as well as inside. Walking, as mentioned in Chapter 6, can not only help reduce soreness and achiness, but also speeds recovery and can provide much-needed aerobic exercise.

I advise walking a minimum of half an hour to an hour every day, though during your first days at home you need not necessarily do all of your walking in one stretch.

"I was walking from the day I got home," says Rachel. "At first, I would just walk the length of my apartment. And then, I remember venturing out as a monumental time. Every day I would go outside with somebody. It was always a supervised walk with either one of my parents or my husband. I remember going up and down stairs within the first few days, and that was really kind of neat."

Walking a minimum of 30 minutes a day is the only exercise I specifically ask patients to do upon discharge from the hospital, but I also emphasize a return as soon as possible to other aerobic physical activity. Exercising will likely cause some pain at first, since the muscles around your back and in your legs will have lost some strength through disuse. But in general, the more you do it, the more comfortable it will become and the better you will feel. (If exercising causes dizziness or *excessive* pain, you should stop and try again later.) Any type of aerobic exercise will advance your recovery: brisk walking, using a treadmill, a Stairmaster, or a Nordic track, riding an exercise bicycle. Once the incision has completely healed, generally two weeks or so after surgery, you can do aerobic exercise—walking or swimming—in a swimming pool.

"Swimming, now that was a challenge," says Arlene. "I went to a town pool here, and I could feel—I knew I had something in my back that I hadn't had before. I had always been a swimmer. But I went to take that first stroke and I thought, 'Oh, dear God, I'm going to sink.' Now, whether that was just in my mind or what, I don't know. But I did feel that right away, though I don't feel it anymore. But it's a little tough because I can tell where he fused me. The old mobility is not there."

When patients come to see me for their first postoperative office visit, one month after surgery, I usually put them on a more formal exercise and/or physical therapy program. Sometimes I tell patients to get a set of light weights and a videotape of light-impact aerobics and use that program. Patients who want or need a more formal, structured program I send to physical therapy, where they first learn exercises intended to restore range of motion in the thoracolumbar spine, the hips, the legs, etc. The physical therapist also works with patients on improving aerobic conditioning. Gradually, as you feel better, the therapist will work up to resistive work with weights, building muscle strength throughout the legs, back, and arms. After six months or so, you can probably do a full workout without any restrictions.

As far as other activities of daily living go, I now adopt a fairly laissez-faire attitude. As soon as you feel comfortable doing something, go ahead and do it. I used to tell patients not to drive a car until after the first postoperative office visit one month later, but now I say that if they feel up to it, they can take short rides in their neighborhood or community within a few weeks. I still would not recommend long car rides, because it forces people to remain in basically the same position for too long a time.

You may find that you can't do everything you want to do right away, and you may need to figure out some ingenious ways to manage on your own during the times when you don't have help. Betty had her husband buy her a "grabber," a small claw at the end of a 24-inch stick, with which she could pick things up when they fell without having to bend or stoop. Betty also came up with a system that allowed her to begin cooking for her family about ten days after getting home. "I lined my counters with my pots and pans because when I had to cook, I couldn't bend down to the bottom cabinets to get them out," she explains. "So if I knew what I was cooking that night, I would have my husband take everything out and set it up. As long as everything was at a good level, I could do what I had to do."

In general, postsurgical patients' instrumentation is very solidly fixed and there is little need to worry about hardware coming apart as a result of their level of activity. Nevertheless, you should be wary of putting yourself in any position where you might take a bad fall or become involved in a high-speed accident. For at least the first six months, it would be wise to avoid snow skiing, water skiing, housepainting, stock-car racing, skydiving, tightrope walking, and pole-vaulting—which I always make a point of adding to this list since, as I mentioned earlier, a patient sent me a picture of himself pole-vaulting in a school track meet just four months after his operation.

In most cases, the more active you are during this initial recovery period, the easier activities will become and the faster you will recuperate. Gradually, over the course of the first few weeks at home, you should increase your level of activities until you have returned to your presurgical level—or better!

Sex and Pregnancy

Most adults who have had scoliosis surgery also wonder about sexual relations. I tell my patients that they can resume sexual activity whenever they feel comfortable doing so. Some patients undoubtedly have sex the first night they go home. Others may wait until their follow-up X-rays show that fusion has completely healed, six months or a year after surgery, before asking when they can start having sex again.

"The first time I had sex after the surgery was really kind of monumental," Rachel recalls. "That was precarious. I think my husband was very nervous, but it was just very delicate. I had lost a lot of weight, and I'm small to start out with. I was a little wraith and very fragile. If I remember, it was only two weeks after I got home. But it was fine. It was nice doing that again. And it was a cause for celebration."

When you resume sexual relations, use your own judgment regarding sexual positions and sexual activities. As long as you feel comfortable, there are no sexual positions that you cannot enjoy. A woman might find it easier in the beginning to be on top during sex rather than lying underneath with her partner's weight on top. A heterosexual man might also find it more comfortable to have his partner on top so that he won't have to do all the thrusting, which might be painful for him at first. Finally, since those who wear postoperative braces only need to wear them during upright activities, unless you are upright you will not need to keep the brace on during sexual activity.

If you have sex during the first six months after surgery, I strongly recommend using appropriate birth-control methods to avoid pregnancy. In cautioning against pregnancy following scoliosis surgery, I am concerned with the possible impact of pregnancy on an incomplete fusion. Even the most severe cases of scoliosis have little documented effect on either a pregnancy or the development of a fetus. To have a negative impact on the developing fetus, a woman would have to have a very large curve (approaching 100 degrees) and severe restrictive lung disease as a result. Since this condition might interfere with the oxygenation of the blood, the fetus might suffer damage from inadequate oxygen supply. However, not only are curves of this size exceedingly rare today, but even then, I have neither seen nor heard of any cases that document this. So you need not worry about the effect of scoliosis on your baby.

As for the pregnancy itself, scoliosis might add to the back pain that pregnancy can produce. However, all women, with or without scoliosis, run the risk of back pain with pregnancy. The best predictor of back pain during pregnancy is not the presence of scoliosis, but rather a history of back pain during previous pregnancies. Among the scoliosis patients I have treated who later became pregnant, none to my knowledge developed significant or disabling back pain during their pregnancies.

During labor and delivery, a long fusion of the lumbar spine (involving vertebrae lower than L4) might interfere with the anesthetist's ability to administer epidural anesthesia, which is administered through a catheter that passes through the vertebrae into the lower spinal canal. Fusing low lumbar vertebrae into a solid bone can block access to the spinal canal. But since very few fusions go below L4, there is usually room for the needle to pass below this vertebra. So I encourage my patients (and their obstetrical anesthetists) not to rule out an epidural until they first try. Unless they've had a long lumbar fusion, most of those who do will find that they can have an epidural.

Although scoliosis and scoliosis surgery have a minimal impact on future pregnancies, pregnancy has an unpredictable effect on scoliosis. Some but not all curves worsen as a result of pregnancy. What aspect of pregnancy contributes to curve progression and why it does not exercise the same influence on all women with scoliosis are unknown. The extra weight of pregnancy or perhaps the relaxation of tissues due to hormonal changes that allow the birth canal to open may contribute to progression. But no one really knows. All we do know is that some women do have a risk of curve progression during pregnancy.

Pregnancy may also have an adverse impact on spinal-fusion surgery that has not yet fully healed. Since pregnancy puts an additional strain on the back, again, I encourage scoliosis patients to wait six months after surgery before trying to get pregnant. Although that time period is somewhat arbitrary, I would prefer that patients have a reasonably solid fusion before putting it to the test of a pregnancy. Several of my patients, including Karin, have gotten pregnant earlier than six months after surgery. Fortunately, none of them had any problems with their pregnancy and all went on to solid fusions. Despite their happy endings, though, I would not recommend pregnancy during the initial postoperative period.

"After having tried for years and not getting pregnant, including two months of in vitro that didn't work, I got pregnant six weeks after surgery. Truly that had to be the closest thing to immaculate conception," Karin says with a laugh. "My husband was afraid to come near me. And I had no problem with the pregnancy. I had to stop doing certain back-strengthening exercises that were inappropriate for the early months of a pregnancy, when you're trying to be very careful you don't lose the baby. But I was far enough along with those exercises that it didn't matter. I truly had an easy, nonproblematical pregnancy. If anything, I had less trouble with back pain than I did with my first pregnancy. I was more comfortable. And I was lucky that I didn't have an X-ray when I shouldn't have an X-ray. I had an X-ray one month after surgery, and by the time I came back two months later, I was pregnant. And then I had an X-ray as soon as I could after the delivery and everything had fused fine. I count myself very lucky in every sense of the word."

Coping with Postoperative Pain

"Even three weeks after I came home," Alison recalls, "the pain was still quite great and that was surprising. I couldn't walk very far without a lot of pain, and I used to wait for the pain to come on, it was so tremendous. Just getting back into life for someone who was my age, thirty-seven if you want to know, took time. It was surprisingly difficult."

All patients will have pain when they get home. Certain activities and exercises will cause pain, and you will also probably feel some pain just sitting or lying down. The amount of pain depends upon such factors as age and the procedure that was performed. Thoracoplasties tend to cause a little more postoperative pain. But the extent of pain also varies considerably from patient to patient, making it hard to predict exactly how much pain *you* will feel. Nevertheless, you should be prepared for the fact that you will not be pain-free the day you leave the hospital.

Incisional pain goes away fairly quickly, especially among adolescents, who tend to recover much faster than adults. Pain from the graft site and from thoracoplasty, if performed, tends to be more persistent, but even this pain tends to decrease over time. As mentioned in Chapter 6, a graph of the amount of post-surgical pain you will feel would look more like a mountain range than a steadily sloping hill. A few weeks after coming home, you may be pain-free for several days in a row, only to have a recurrence of postsurgical back pain—or, even more discouraging, a recurrence of *pre*surgical back pain.

Even if scoliosis surgery has successfully treated your pain problem, you may occasionally have a recurrence of old back pain. "We planned to celebrate New Year's Eve, which was about seven weeks after my surgery," Rachel remembers. "Of course, we couldn't make too much of an evening of it, but we went to the movies and dinner. And I had a recurrence of the old backache, not the new pain that I had as a direct result of the surgery but the exact kind of backache that I had felt prior to the surgery. And I panicked, thinking, 'Shoot, I've gone through all this and I still have this old backache.'"

Though your spine may be much straighter after surgery, the muscles around the spine will not immediately adjust to this correction. Many postsurgical pain problems originate in these muscles, rather than in the spine itself. Since it takes time for these muscles to accommodate themselves to the changes in your spine, for a while they will tend to hurt the way they did prior to surgery. Physical therapy and exercise can often help eliminate any recurring pain by gradually building up the strength of the muscles surrounding the spine. Your physical therapist will train the muscles to become better equipped to handle not only everyday tasks but also any additional workload they need to bear as a result of the fusion. "I did take some physical therapy for pain management and muscle strengthening, which I was really happy about," Rachel says. "The pain occurred maybe once or twice in early January. But since then, I've never felt a shred of pain."

"I was lucky to be able to structure my life to leave time to do my physical therapy," Karin says. "And that helped a lot, just in recuperating pretty quickly. It helped me get on with my life faster, being conscientious about physical therapy."

In addition to setting aside the time for physical therapy, you can ease postsurgical pain through drugs. When you return home from the hospital, you will almost certainly have a prescription for a narcotic pain medication, though some patients are down to just Tylenol by the time of discharge. Most teen-agers, because they recover quickly and their pain tends to diminish relatively soon after surgery, will have a prescription only for codeine or Tylenol-3, which has codeine in it. Again, it is important to remember that children do have pain, just as adults do, and care should be taken not to *under*medicate them. Most teenagers bounce back from surgery very quickly, and may therefore need to take analgesics regularly for only a week or so after getting home. Susannah took Tylenol-3 three times a day for the first three or four days and then just once a day for another three or four days. If the pain occasionally recurs, however, parents should not be reluctant to let their children take codeine to help manage their pain.

Since adults generally feel more severe pain and take longer to recover from surgery, they may need a stronger painkiller than Tylenol-3. Adults also tend to remain on the narcotics for longer than children. Severe postoperative pain may be resolved only through pain medications, so you should take them as needed. Nevertheless, I would encourage you to get off prescription painkillers as soon as you can. Since anyone who takes narcotics for an extended period of time runs the risk of addiction, take care not to depend too much on your pain medication to deal with every ache and twinge. Physical therapy, exercise, stretching, relaxation, and meditation help manage pain without the risk of addiction.

Most adult scoliosis patients remain on narcotics for up to a month after surgery. Usually, by the time my patients come for their first postoperative office visit one month after surgery, they are either no longer taking narcotics at all or perhaps taking one only at night to help them sleep. Indeed, I encourage my patients to stop taking prescription painkillers by their first postoperative visit. I usually write a prescription that lasts for a month after discharge. After that, I will generally *not* renew the prescription.

"I tried to get off the Percocet as fast as I could," Karin says. "After a few days home, I wasn't taking Percocet except at night. The one thing my doctor said was to not take a fall, and I just felt a little looped on those things. I felt steadier on my feet without them."

Getting off prescription narcotics will also help normalize your bowel functioning. As mentioned earlier, codeine tends to cause constipation. For this reason, some patients need regular enemas in the first few weeks at home to flush their systems out. Once you're off the painkillers your bowels will soon return to normal.

Once you have stopped taking prescription narcotics, you can probably manage any pain that arises with Tylenol, which is not an anti-inflammatory, but strictly an analgesic—a pain pill. Some literature suggests that nonsteroidal anti-inflammatory medications (aspirin, Motrin, Advil, Alleve, etc.) may interfere with the process of fusion, so you should *avoid taking nonsteroidal anti-inflammatories* for at least three months after surgery.

No matter how much pain you feel in the initial weeks after surgery, recognize that this painful process of recovery does have an end. If pain motivated you to seek surgical treatment in the first place, chances are very good that this original chronic and severe back pain will become occasional, or even rare, and less intense. And the pain caused by the surgery itself will almost definitely pass. Just listen to what these three patients have to say about their pain today:

"I can't believe, even though it's only been six months, that I used to feel that way," says Alison. "How very rapidly I lost what in essence was a very big part of my life: pain. I no longer look for it. I'm just surprised that I don't have it anymore and that I don't even think about pain."

"What the surgery has done for me is incredible," says Arlene. "Before surgery my doctor told me my chances of being pain-free would be about seventy percent. Well, I would say I'm almost ninety percent better. With the pain that I was experiencing before I had the surgery, there was no question in my mind that I'd either end up paralyzed because of the condition or end up in a wheelchair. I have none of that pain now, none of it."

"I can't tell you how great it's been," Rachel agrees. "I'm perfectly straight now, never had a day of pain after the effects of the surgery wore off, and I've been totally fine. I'm thirty-one now. I had the surgery when I was twenty-nine, and it's been great, fantastic!"

Will You Feel the Hardware Inside You?

When patients first learn that scoliosis surgery involves the implantation of metal rods to support the spine in its corrected position, most want to know how it will feel to have these rods inside them. In general, patients do not feel the rods themselves. The rods do not come into contact with any nerve endings and should therefore cause no sensation in and of themselves. Yet some patients do insist that they can feel the rods: "I don't really have any problems with it," says Arlene, "but I can tell you this. I know when it's going to rain. And on a cold day, I know those rods are in my back."

Patients more commonly feel the hardware that holds the rods in place rather than the rods themselves. Especially when attached to the spine posteriorly, hooks or clamps can sometimes be prominent. They may poke against the inside of the skin on your back and can sometimes cause local but intense pain when touched. Your surgeon will attempt to place these hooks and clamps in ways that minimize their prominence and reduce the incidence of pain. In some cases, however, despite the surgeon's best efforts, this hardware becomes problematic.

"The doctors tell you that you're not going to feel the rods," Betty says skeptically. "Maybe I don't feel the rods, but I sure as heck felt all the rest of the hardware. I had one hook very close to the surface of my spine and I could never sit back in a chair because it stabbed me and when it happened I got a feeling like an electrical shock. And if somebody bumped into me or if somebody put their hand around me and touched me in that one spot, it was incredibly painful."

Once the bone has fused and healed, the instrumentation is no longer necessary, but scoliosis surgeons do not routinely take the hardware out because it would require another operation. However, if the hardware is too prominent, if it breaks or loosens and no longer supports the incomplete fusion, and especially if it causes pain, the surgeon may need to perform a second operation to remove the hardware. Betty had her hardware removed after the top crossbar that links the two rods broke. "I definitely felt that there was movement," she explains, "and I felt very uncomfortable where the hooks were. So it was worth it to me to have the surgery."

Not all broken hardware needs to be surgically removed. Betty had surgery not just because the hardware had broken but because it led to increased pain and discomfort. If your spine has completely healed and you have a piece of broken hardware that is painful, then it needs to be taken out. If your spine has not yet fused and broken hardware has allowed a recurrence of the deformity, the hardware needs to be replaced, often after additional surgical reconstruction. But if an X-ray shows a piece of broken hardware, and yet you look fine and feel fine and have no symptoms from the broken hardware, your orthopedist should leave the hardware alone.

Whether or not you feel the rods and the other hardware, you will almost definitely feel the impact of the rods, and the fusion that the rods protect, in a loss of some mobility. The rods, and eventually the fusion, will prevent you from moving the spine in the fused area. This is one of the primary goals of the surgery. When your spine was flexible and mobile, it curved progressively. By fixing part of the spine in place, this curvature can be corrected and arrested. To achieve this correction, however, you must sacrifice a certain degree of mobility. Lumbar fusions can produce notable stiffness and loss of mobility. The thoracic spine—where most scoliotic curves are located—is fortunately involved in very few essential back movements, so the loss of mobility owing to thoracic fusions is hardly noticed. Karin had a selective thoracic fusion from T4 to T12. Now, she says, "I think I'm a little more restricted. I don't think I can bend as far from side to side, but it's not something I really do anyway unless I'm doing side-bending exercises. For bending over, I don't feel restricted at all, though I did feel it for a time when I was recuperating from the surgery. Now I bend down and pick up my child twenty-two hundred times a day. I lug around a twenty-five-pound baby half the day. My *arms* might get sore, but not my back."

Most scoliosis patients would gladly sacrifice some movement in order to have their spine corrected. If you have opted for surgical intervention because of persistent pain, that pain no doubt imposes more restrictions on your movement and activities than the stiffness of a fused spine will. Though you may lose a significant degree of mobility, particularly if you undergo a lumbar fusion, this loss should not prevent you from participating in any physical activities you enjoy.

Back to Normal

"I remember feeling really good for the first time about six weeks after my surgery," says Rachel. "I'd gone Christmas shopping with my mother. I was away from the house for two hours, and even though I returned absolutely exhausted and in pain, I just felt so liberated. It was the first time I remember feeling really kind of back to normal."

A month after your discharge from the hospital, you will need to see your orthopedist and obtain a new set of X-rays. I generally order two X-rays during follow-ups: an A-P and a lateral to check the status of the fusion and make sure everything remains intact. By comparing these X-rays with those taken immediately after the operation, your orthopedist can see whether the spine or the instrumentation has shifted at all.

At this point, most teenagers are ready to go back to school; some kids recover so quickly that they want to return to school even earlier. I used to dissuade teenagers from going back to school until after I had a chance to see them. But today, if a patient's parents call me two weeks after discharge and tell me the child feels great and wants to go back to school, I say fine, go ahead. I trust my patients to know when they're ready, and I don't believe that they need to be treated like delicate flowers just because they underwent surgery.

Adults generally need a little longer time to recuperate before being ready to go back to work. "I went back to work four months after the operation," remembers Arlene, who does clerical work in a doctor's office. "I couldn't do any lifting or any of that, but I went back full time right away. Once in a while, there was a lot of discomfort in the muscles. But I did fine." Depending upon the nature of your work, you may be ready to go back within six weeks to three months, although some patients, and some jobs, demand more recovery time. If you had a circumferential fusion (front and back surgery), you might need six months at home before returning to work.

By your second postoperative visit, three months after surgery, you will probably be feeling much more comfortable. Most patients feel little or no pain by this point and have discontinued or reduced to a bare minimum the use of pain medications. Usually by this time, patients are ready and willing to do anything. I tell patients that at this point, they can be fully active except for those activities in which they might take a bad fall.

"At four months I would say I felt like I had progressed quite a bit," Alison remembers. "At five and a half months, you realize that you can start living a normal life. I had had a lot of pain before surgery, and then five, six months later I realized that this is more or less what other people feel like. You're normal, and *that* was strange. Because in a funny way, you still don't know what normal people are like. You have really no sensation of what it is to be normal. I guess I hadn't had that since I was eleven years old."

After six months, when you visit your orthopedist for the third time, you can do absolutely anything—all activities without restrictions of any kind—as long as your X-rays look good. You can ski or sky-dive, whatever you want to do. Although complete fusion usually takes between six months and a year, I let my patients be fully active after six months because by this time, the fusion has progressed to a significant degree. (If it has not healed within a year after surgery, it probably will not heal and may require revision surgery.) After this visit, I ask patients to come back and get a new set of X-rays every year for the next five years or so to check on the status of the fusion and the degree of curvature. Assuming that the fusion heals properly and no further problems arise, I then say good-bye and wish my patients all the best.

For most people, successful scoliosis surgery results in an emotional transformation as well as a physical one. Once you have faced and survived major surgery, you may feel you can survive anything, and other problems often seem less important. You may concern yourself less with little worries and hardships and appreciate little joys more. Life may seem sweeter. In any case, surgery will change you in tangible and intangible ways.

"I really did see my life in a very different way," says Susannah, "because I remembered what it felt like not to have to worry about anything big. So it's definitely been a major part of my life. I think I had to deal with some very scary issues and fears at a very young age, and it *did* make me appreciate life and health a lot more than I think some of my peers did. So in a weird way, I'm glad it happened."

CHAPTER EIGHT

Degenerative

Scoliosis

IN THE PAST TWO DECADES, ORTHOPEDISTS HAVE increasingly recognized a form of scoliosis that does not follow the same developmental pattern as other scolioses. Unlike most idiopathic as well as congenital and neuromuscular scolioses, this newly identified scoliosis does not appear during early childhood or adolescence and then progress as the body physically matures. Instead, this type of scoliosis, known as *degenerative scoliosis*, develops in a previously straight spine during adult life, some time *after* the cessation of growth. Typically, degenerative scoliosis develops as a result of degenerative changes that occur in the spine. As discs wear out and/or the facet joints become arthritic as part of the aging process, the spine begins to lose stability. As a result of this instability, spinal curves may develop.

In the coming decades, degenerative scoliosis will become an increasingly common disorder. Since disc degeneration and arthritis of the joints occur primarily as a result of aging, people who develop degenerative scoliosis tend to be much older than those who develop other scolioses. As more people live to older ages, it makes sense that the incidence of degenerative scoliosis will increase as well.

Like idiopathic scolioses, degenerative scoliosis occurs more commonly in women than in men. Although the relationship remains unclear, degenerative scoliosis may have some connection to osteoporosis, a condition (also more common among women) marked by brittle or porous bones resulting from the loss of calcium. Among women, the incidence of degenerative scoliosis and the rate of curve progression rises rapidly around the time of menopause, a time also associated with the onset of osteoporosis. Among patients with idiopathic scoliosis, the size of curves also increases dramatically during menopause. Clearly, the onset of osteoporosis and the reduction in hormone levels brought on by menopause, if not the direct cause of degenerative scoliosis, are at least linked to the progression of all kinds of scoliosis, and perhaps also to the onset of degenerative scoliosis. As a group, those with degenerative scoliosis will generally also have problems with osteoporosis. (If osteoporosis is a significant problem for you, your orthopedist should probably refer you to an appropriate specialist to evaluate you for any weakness of the bony skeleton caused by osteoporosis and for appropriate medical management of such weakness.)

Many older adults today remain much more active than their predecessors just a generation ago, and this puts more demands on their spines. Aging and day-to-day activity cause wear and tear in the spine. Discs gradually degenerate, undergoing changes in their chemical structure. Discs dry out and, like sponges, shrink as they lose fluid content. The annulus, the fibrous cartilage ring that surrounds the pulpy center of a disc, may tear. This degeneration can lead to what I call disc disorganization, or the inability of the discs and facet joints to perform their proper mechanical function. When a disc degenerates it can cause malalignment of the vertebra above it. As a result of the changes in the disc, the vertebra may rotate and slide off the vertebra below it, a condition known as lateral listhesis or rotatory subluxation.

Idiopathic curves also progress as a result of disc degeneration, so the distinction between true degenerative scoliosis and idiopathic scoliosis that degenerates with age is not always clear. The latter is, however, a different entity from true degenerative scoliosis. A person may have had an idiopathic scoliosis that was not all that large and therefore went undiagnosed earlier. As a result of degenerative changes in the spine, the curve may then progress significantly in the older adult.

Degenerative scoliosis does have a number of distinguishing characteristics that differentiate it from idiopathic scoliosis. For instance, the curvatures in a true degenerative scoliosis seldom become very large. Typically, they range from 15 degrees to 40 degrees, with very few curves ever exceeding 50 degrees. Degenerative curves also tend to be shorter, involving fewer vertebrae, than idiopathic curves. Curve location provides another clue to help identify the presence of degenerative scoliosis. Typical degenerative curves are lumbar or thoracolumbar—the apex is at the junction between the thoracic and lumbar spines. Indeed, a degenerative curve may exist entirely within the lumbosacral spine, a location never seen with idiopathic scoliosis.

Degenerative scoliosis is also more commonly associated with sagittal plane problems than idiopathic scoliosis, though the latter can also lead to sagittal abnormalities. Since the curves it causes are not generally located in the thoracic spine, thoracic kyphosis is not usually a significant problem with degenerative scoliosis. However, it often does lead to problems with lumbar lordosis. The discs account for about one-fourth of the height of the vertebral column. As the discs degenerate and collapse, narrow, and settle, the front of the spine loses height. The lumbar spine is normally lordotic: Viewed from the side, it curves forward. Therefore the front of the lumbar spine, on the convex side of this lordotic curve, is longer than the back of the lumbar spine, the concavity of the curve. When the lumbar spine becomes shorter in the front because of the narrowing and collapse of discs, it loses normal lordosis. Disc degeneration and disorganization can thus produce a flattening of the lumbar spine and a loss of normal sagittal contouring, which can in turn lead to the development of secondary symptoms. Typically, sagittal balance becomes impaired, causing the person to pitch forward. That's why so many older people walk with straight backs and tend to pitch slightly forward.

Degenerative scolioses also tend to involve less vertebral rotation than idiopathic scolioses. Disc degeneration generally causes a more asymmetrical collapse of the spinal column, but seldom causes as much rotation as idiopathic scoliosis.

Despite these differences between idiopathic scoliosis and degenerative scoliosis, your orthopedist may not be able to say with certainty which kind of scoliosis you have. For one thing, you may not know whether or not you had a curve when you were younger. Some patients who seem to have idiopathic curves that have degenerated with age nonetheless insist that their spines have always been perfectly straight. Yet their X-rays may show a large curve with a lot of rotation, one that doesn't look like a simple degenerative curve. Whether or not the orthopedist knows what to call it, though, the treatment protocol (see below) will be the same.

Since degenerative curves are not generally large, the main symptom that causes people with degenerative scoliosis to seek treatment is pain. Primarily because of the arthritic changes in the back, people with degenerative scoliosis develop severe back pain. Back pain may also result from malalignment, which heightens the work demands on the back muscles as they attempt to maintain an erect posture. Since the most severe cases of flat-back that result from degenerative scoliosis tend to pitch people forward, they require individuals to flex their hips and knees in order to stand erect. For this reason, these patients experience a lot of leg fatigue and pain.

People with degenerative scoliosis who have milder flat-backs will also typically have leg pain. This leg pain comes as a result of nerve-root entrapment caused by the disc collapse, disc degeneration, or disc disorganization, especially the lateral slippage of vertebrae. A healthy disc may start out at about a centimeter in height, but degenerative changes can cut this in half. This shrinkage leaves less room for the nerves in the section of the spinal canal adjacent to this collapsed disc. This narrowing or constriction of the spinal canal is known as *spinal stenosis*, a condition that often leads to nerve-root entrapment.

Nerve-root entrapment does not always result from disc collapse. More commonly, it results from arthritic changes in the facet joints. People with this type of spinal stenosis, called developmental spinal stenosis, start out with a relatively normal spinal canal. Arthritis causes the facet joints of the spine to become enlarged, not unlike big arthritic knuckles. Directly underneath these facet joints run nerve roots of the spine as they exit the spinal canal. As arthritic facet joints enlarge, they can reduce the amount of space available in the spinal canal and thus impinge on these nerve roots, causing nerve-root entrapment.

Spinal stenosis can also result from the progressive thickening of the ligamentum flavum, a ligament in the spine. As the ligamentum flavum thickens, it narrows the space available for the nerves. In most cases, spinal stenosis results from a combination of all of these factors.

Spinal stenosis does occur in some idiopathic scolioses, but much less commonly. Entirely separate from scoliosis, it can also develop in people who do not have scoliosis. When spinal stenosis is associated with scoliotic curves, however, it usually indicates the presence of degenerative scoliosis.

During a patient's initial history and physical, certain complaints generally point to the presence of spinal stenosis. The most common complaint associated with spinal stenosis is called *spinal claudication*, a cramping that people get in their calves because of nerve entrapment. Spinal claudication makes walking extremely difficult and painful. In milder cases, the patient may be able to walk several blocks before cramping occurs. In more severe cases, though, cramps may start after just a half a block. Unlike cramps associated with vascular claudication, a condition caused by inadequate blood flow, those associated with spinal claudication do not stop when the individual stops walking. Typically, the person will need to sit down or sometimes lean forward in order to relieve the pain. Although spinal stenosis may also be associated with numbness, tingling, or occasional weakness, spinal claudication is its most characteristic symptom.

A thorough medical history and physical exam should reveal whether you have these symptoms characteristic of spinal stenosis and degenerative scoliosis. The next step is obtaining a set of X-rays, especially anteroposterior X-rays, which reveal the presence of any lateral scoliotic curves, and lateral X-rays, which show the extent of your flat-back. If the findings of the history, physical, and X-rays are inconsistent or confusing, raising doubts as to whether you have a spinal stenosis or some other back problem, your doctor will probably order electrical studies and/or vascular studies—an ultrasound study of the blood vessels—to help arrive at a more precise diagnosis. On the other hand, if the findings of your history, physical, and X-rays are consistent with a diagnosis of degenerative scoliosis and spinal stenosis, your doctor will probably order an additional radiographic diagnostic study to confirm it. This consists of either computerized axial tomography (a CAT scan), magnetic resonance imaging (MRI), or a myelogram, obtained by injecting dye into the spinal canal prior to taking X-rays and performing a CAT scan, which employs X-ray sweeps to produce vividly detailed cross-sectional images of the spine.

Although the combination of a myelogram and a CAT scan provide more detailed and useful information, I sometimes order an MRI first simply because it is not invasive and can be performed on an outpatient basis. The MRI, a magnetic device linked to a computer, gives a three-dimensional image of the inside of the body. To undergo an MRI, you lie on a retractable shelf, which is slid back into the machine with you on it. You find yourself enclosed in a small, bright, white tube not much larger than your body, a situation that some find extremely claustrophobic. You must lie with your arms at your sides and not move until the procedure has been completed. When the machine is activated, it makes a lot of noise, which can frighten some people. (Many facilities now offer earphones, allowing the patient to listen to music during the MRI.) The MRI is perfectly safe, however, presenting no known health hazards, except for one: Since they create images through the generation of a strong magnetic field, those with cardiac pacemakers or other implanted metal-containing devices should *not* get an MRI. After about 45 minutes of this deafening noise and stillness, the machine will stop operating and the shelf will be slid back out. The capabilities of MRIs have improved in recent years, and they now provide the best possible evaluation of the nutritional status of discs—water content, etc.—and therefore of disc degeneration itself.

Although MRIs provide valuable information on disc degeneration, I often need a more complete picture of bone detail than they can offer. Spinal stenosis more commonly stems from arthritic enlargement of the spine's bony elements (for example, overly large facet joints) than from disc degeneration, so I frequently order myelograms combined with a CAT scan, which provide a better look at bone detail. The dye injected into the spinal canal for a myelogram provides a strong contrast with bony elements that cause nerve-root compression, and thus provide a powerful indication of the site of nerve-root compression.

A myelogram and a postmyelographic CAT scan provide the best test available for spinal stenosis associated with degenerative scoliosis. The myelogram provides a road map of the neural networks. The map displays a main route, the big sac of nerves, and lots of little branches, the nerve roots that come off at every level of the spine. By studying the CAT-scan monitor, the doctor can quickly see whether any nerve-root compression exists. Compression will prevent the nerve from filling properly with the dye, so if the doctor sees an area where dye should be, but isn't, it indicates some degree of stenosis. If nerve-root compression does exist, the CAT scan helps the doctor determine where it occurs, what causes it, and what the offending structures are.

A myelogram is done by a radiologist. You receive a local anesthesia, and perhaps a mild sedative if you need it, but remain awake throughout this procedure. The radiologist inserts a thin needle into your lower back, which passes through the muscle and into the spinal canal. When the needle passes through the sac that surrounds all the nerves and holds the spinal fluid, a small amount of spinal fluid comes back through the needle and into the syringe. This is the sign for the radiologist to inject a barium-based dye into the spinal fluid and remove the needle. Now the spinal fluid will show up on regular X-rays, which can be made with the spine in various positions. The radiologist will then send you to a CAT-scanning unit, where you will undergo a CAT scan. Although the machine looks similar to an MRI machine, important differences do exist. Most people find CAT scans much easier to tolerate than MRIs because a CAT scan does not enclose your whole body but leaves your head and neck free, so you are less likely to get claustrophobic. CAT scans do expose patients to X-rays, and the objective of obtaining a three-dimensional image makes shielding impossible. Yet unlike standard X-rays, which may be required on a regular basis, CAT scans seldom need to be performed more than once.

Today, a myelogram is a fairly painless and problem-free procedure. Occasionally, a person may get a headache from a myelogram if a little spinal-fluid leak develops afterward, or perhaps a little nausea or leg pain or cramping. But in most cases, patients suffer no ill effects, undergoing the procedure on an outpatient basis and leaving the hospital the same day.

Treatment for Degenerative Scoliosis and Spinal Stenosis

Once your history, physical, X-rays, and other diagnostic tests have pointed to a diagnosis of degenerative scoliosis, you and your orthopedist will need to decide on an appropriate treatment. The type of treatment depends on the severity of your symptoms. If you have degenerative scoliosis and some back pain, your symptoms will initially be treated the same way back pain is treated in other patients: through anti-inflammatory medications, exercise, physical therapy, and external back supports. Your doctor will probably give you some medicine to reduce the inflammation caused by the arthritic changes in your back. You might also be put on an exercise program designed to strengthen your abdominal muscles and your back muscles. Your doctor might also send you to a physical therapist, who will teach you how to strengthen your muscles and increase your resistance to pain as well as help you to stretch. Most people who have pain associated with degenerative scoliosis need a stretching program to overcome tightness in the hamstrings or hip flexors, which can contribute to back pain. Finally, if you have acute symptoms perhaps associated with a specific injury, your doctor may give you an external back support to ease the demands on your back muscles, and hence your pain. Many people with degenerative scoliosis respond very well to these simple recommendations and require no further treatment.

If you do not respond to these treatments, however, you may require surgery. The main, and perhaps *only*, indication for surgical treatment of degenerative scoliosis is *pain*: chronic and severe pain that proves unresponsive to nonoperative treatment. You might have back pain, leg pain, or both. Since pain is the primary symptom that warrants surgery for degenerative scoliosis, the decision about whether or not to operate at all is *always* an elective, quality-of-life decision on the part of the patient. The shape of the back or extent of the deformity *do not* necessarily indicate that surgery is appropriate. A patient may have the worst-looking back around, but if she is not disabled by pain, there's probably no need for surgery.

Weighing the pain factor depends on how you define disability. If your pain incapacitates you at work or inhibits you from your favorite pursuits—playing tennis or going to the movies a couple of times a week—or if you can only walk one or two blocks before you have to stop and sit, you clearly suffer from a loss of function. But you may regard these as inconveniences or annoyances rather than a disability. If you want to avoid a big operation, you may be willing to accept these limitations on your functioning. On the other hand, you may decide that if a reasonable alternative exists that would allow you to walk more comfortably and be more active and do more things, then you might want to pursue that.

Only those who are disabled as a result of the pain associated with degenerative scoliosis and/or spinal stenosis become candidates for surgical treatment. The magnitude of the scoliotic curve rarely plays any part in this decision. Indeed, the degenerative curves of most people who choose surgical treatment are of a magnitude that would seldom indicate surgery in a person with idiopathic scoliosis. It is the presence and persistence of pain associated with these small degenerative curves that indicate the need for surgery.

If you have decided to go ahead with surgery, your surgeon may ask you to undergo a test known as *lumbar discography*. Your orthopedist will want to fuse as few vertebral levels as possible, so it is important to find out which discs are actually causing pain. Discs degenerate naturally as a consequence of aging, and most degenerated discs do *not* cause pain. So if your X-ray shows that you have degenerative scoliosis and a great number of degenerated discs, your doctor will want to know specifically which discs, at what levels, are really responsible for the pain. Will the surgeon need to fuse the levels above and below every degenerated disc? Or might some of those degenerative levels be entirely unrelated to your pain?

Lumbar discography can help answer these questions. Discography is a provocative and extremely unpleasant procedure, but it can provide essential information that your doctor needs to make a decision regarding what vertebral levels to include in the fusion. The procedure must be done on each degenerated disc, to establish whether or not it causes pain similar to the pain chronically experienced by the patient. To perform the test, the doctor inserts a needle into the disc itself and injects a fluid—usually a dye, because on an X-ray, it provides a better idea of the form and structure of the disc—to pressurize the disc. The doctor will want to know, with the injection of each disc, does it cause pain? If so, how severe is it? Is the pain similar in degree, location, and radiation to the pain that you get on an everyday basis? This information is more important than the form and structure of the disc.

Although a description of lumbar discography may sound sadistic, the information gained through this test helps the doctor determine how extensive the operation will need to be. Suppose you have a lumbar curve that ends at L3 and you also have some disc degeneration at L4 and L5. Your surgeon may wonder whether the fusion should extend all the way down to the sacrum. Discography might reveal that neither the L5-S1 disc (the one between the L5 vertebra and the sacrum) nor the L4-L5 disc produces pain. In this case, even though they have degenerated, these levels don't need to be fused. The fusion will only need to go down to the L3 vertebra.

The principles of fusion surgery for degenerative scoliosis are the same as those used in treating idiopathic scoliosis (see Chapter 4). In general, however, degenerative scoliosis does not require fusion at as many levels as idiopathic scoliosis. Since degenerative curves tend to be shorter and have less rotation than idiopathic curves, they require shorter fusions.

Most people whose degenerative scoliosis requires surgical treatment need more than simple fusion surgery. Disabling pain in patients with degenerative scoliosis results more from stenosis than from anything else. So surgical treatment needs to focus primarily on stenotic complaints: a lot of leg pain and perhaps some back pain. To correct spinal stenosis, the surgeon often must perform a *lumbar decompression* (also called a lumbar laminectomy). This involves "unroofing" the spinal canal. If you picture the spine as a cylindrical pipe, unroofing it means opening up one side of this cylinder to turn it into a viaduct — a true canal. This opening up is aimed at providing enough space for the nerves. In some cases, the surgeon can decompress the nerves simply by realigning the spine, by correcting the scoliotic curve. If this sufficiently reduces the stenosis in the spinal canal, a laminectomy becomes unnecessary. But if the stenosis results from arthritically enlarged facet joints, realignment of a typically small deformity will not take care of the problem. These patients will require lumbar decompression.

The failure rate of decompression alone to eliminate pain is high among patients who have degenerative scoliosis and spinal stenosis; for this reason your surgeon will also need to fuse your spine. Most fusions used to stabilize and correct degenerative scoliosis can be performed from the back according to the procedures described in Chapter 4. Certain conditions, however, indicate the need for both anterior and posterior surgery. If you need to be fused all the way down to the sacrum, posterior surgery alone runs a very high risk of pseudoarthrosis (failure of fusion). So your doctor will probably want to operate on you from both front and back. If you have a very large degenerative curve and a great deal of imbalance, you will probably also need anterior surgery to loosen up the spine and allow greater correction posteriorly. Most important, if you have a significant degree of sagittal imbalance, you will need anterior surgery to release (by removing discs) and lengthen (by inserting structural bone grafts) the front of the spine, then posterior surgery to compress the back of the spine. Segmental instrumentation, which can be contoured to preserve or restore lumbar lordosis, offers surgeons a valuable tool to help correct degenerative flat-backs.

In addition to the loss of lumbar lordosis, degenerative scoliosis also produces a lateral (side-to-side) curve. However, in most surgical cases involving true degenerative scoliosis, curve correction is not a priority, primarily because curves do not generally get very large. From the standpoint of deformity in degenerative cases, it's much more important to correct the sagittal imbalance than the scoliotic curvature. Treatment of degenerative scoliosis focuses much more on sagittal contouring because that tends to be a major component of the problem. The sagittal concerns raised by idiopathic scoliosis more commonly involve the challenge of maintaining sagittal curves while correcting lateral curves, rather than correcting a significant sagittal deformity. By contrast, degenerative scoliosis almost always leads to sagittal deformities—that is, a loss of lumbar lordosis. For this reason, surgical treatment usually focuses on restoring sagittal balance and spinal stability.

In terms of the choice of internal fixation, your surgeon may have limited options. If the problem that indicated the need for surgery was primarily back pain from a degenerative scoliosis, the surgeon can use hooks, wires, or screws to hold in place the instrumentation that will stabilize the curve. However, if you have had a lumbar laminectomy to decompress the spinal cord and relieve your spinal stenosis, your surgeon cannot fix the segmental instrumentation using either hooks or wires because there's nothing left to which the hooks or wires can be attached. The surgeon will need to use pedicle-screw fixation (see Chapter 4).

For patients with degenerative scoliosis, posterior surgery typically lasts three to five hours and requires about a week of postoperative hospitalization. Front and back surgery of course requires much more time both in the operating room and in the hospital afterward. Depending on the quality of his bone, a patient may need to wear a postoperative brace for three to six months after surgery. Since many patients with degenerative scoliosis also have osteoporosis, they more commonly wear postoperative braces because the instrumentation supporting the spine may itself need some additional support. In most cases, however, the brace is worn only for upright activities, so patients do not have to sleep in it.

Although most risks are minor, the rate of complications following surgery for degenerative scoliosis does tend to be higher than it is for idiopathic patients. This increased risk has more to do with the age of the patients—who are generally in their fifties, sixties, or early seventies, rather than in their twenties or thirties—than anything else.

When people who have degenerative scoliosis reach their mid-seventies or eighties, the risk of complications becomes very high. For this reason, I do not consider patients of this age suitable candidates for surgery and urge them instead to consider any possible alternatives to surgery. Some surgeons will operate on scoliotic patients in their late seventies, but I regard that as pushing the envelope. I believe that the risks of surgery outweigh the potential benefits for patients of this age.

The best option for patients in their late seventies or eighties who have degenerative scoliosis and back pain is probably a custom-made TLSO brace. With this patient population, bracing does not aim to correct the curve or prevent progression, but only to support the patient in an upright position. Unfortunately, many people of this age don't tolerate braces very well. Since older people with scoliosis tend to have very rigid deformities, attempts to squeeze them into a brace can cause intense discomfort. A patient who cannot tolerate a brace may benefit from a lumbar belt, an elasticized cloth belt that can be tightened around the belly. Externally tightening the abdominal muscles works in essentially the same way that strengthening your abdominal muscles with exercise would. Since both provide better support for the back, the back muscles don't have to work quite so hard.

Although these older patients with degenerative scoliosis are difficult to treat, younger patients—those in their fifties to early seventies—can usually be treated quite effectively. Disc degeneration, arthritis, and osteoporosis—and therefore the scoliosis and spinal stenosis they can produce—are natural consequences of aging. But while doctors can do little or nothing to restore the condition of your degenerating discs or to make your arthritis go away, they can often correct your scoliosis and spinal stenosis and thereby ease or eliminate the pain associated with them. Appropriate surgical treatment for degenerative scoliosis will not reverse the process of aging or make you live longer, but it can help you live better and dramatically improve the quality of your life.

CHAPTER NINE

Answers to Commonly Asked Questions

IF YOU OR YOUR CHILD HAS BEEN DIAGNOSED WITH scoliosis, advised to wear a brace, or asked to consider surgery, you no doubt have many questions. I spend a great deal of time with my patients trying to educate them as best I can, answering any questions, doubts, or concerns they may have. The questions generally depend upon the severity of the scoliosis. If your doctor has recommended nothing more than observation, you probably want answers to general questions: what scoliosis is, why it progresses, what conditions might warrant treatment. If your doctor has suggested a brace, your concerns will focus on bracing itself: what it aims to accomplish, how much and how long you will need to wear the brace. Finally, if your doctor has advised surgery, you will have questions concerning the surgery itself and recovery: what the goals of surgery are, how long you will need to be in the hospital, when you can expect to be back on your feet. In this chapter, you will find answers to the questions most commonly asked by my patients. Although I have tried to include all of the questions that commonly come up, if you have any additional questions, be sure to consult your orthopedist.

What is scoliosis?

Scoliosis is a lateral (side-to-side) curvature of the spine. When you look at someone from either the front or the back, the spine should be straight. If it curves at all to the left or right or both ways (forming an S), that's scoliosis.

How much deviation from the straight line is normal in the spine?

None. No scoliosis is normal. However, the diagnosis of scoliosis is made only in the case of curves that measure 10 degrees or more on an X-ray.

Was I born with scoliosis?

Congenital scoliosis, which involves abnormalities in spinal segmentation or failures of spinal formation, by definition results from birth defects. If you have idiopathic scoliosis, which accounts for about five out of six scoliosis diagnoses, you had a straight spine at birth. But as you matured, the spine grew in a crooked fashion.

Will scoliosis go away?

No. Scoliosis does not get better. Scoliosis only stays the same or gets worse. Among some preadolescent children, chiefly 9- and 10-year-olds, the curve may appear to improve for a short period of time, but it always then reverts to its original size or becomes even larger. The *only* reliable way to correct any scoliotic curve is through surgery.

Why does scoliosis progress?

Since curves progress most rapidly during an adolescent's growth spurt and slow down as the chlid reaches skeletal maturity, progression is clearly related to growth. But no one has yet nailed down any specific *causes* of idiopathic curve progression in either children or adults. Among adults, progression may occur simply in reaction to gravity. Structural engineers recognize that any column subjected to a certain amount of force will begin to buckle. In adults who have scoliosis, the force of gravity—weight—is applied to the spinal column, already bent to some degree, over the course of many years. Since a bent column buckles more easily than a straight one, the force of body weight alone may cause further spinal buckling, or curve progression.

Does being overweight affect curve progression?

No documented relationship between weight and curve progression exists, though it makes sense that there might be a connection.

Will becoming pregnant affect curve progression?

Pregnancy has an unpredictable impact on scoliosis. Although orthopedists and the general public alike once thought that pregnancy definitely made curves worse, most recent studies suggest that pregnancy may worsen some curves but leave others unchanged. Since no one can accurately foresee what effect pregnancy will have on any individual's scoliosis, I encourage all women with scoliosis to obtain a new X-ray after each pregnancy. You do not need to avoid pregnancy, but you should be aware of its possible impact on your curve.

Does arthritis have any relationship to scoliosis?

Yes. People who have severe scoliosis will tend to develop spondylosis, or arthritis of the spine, as a result of abnormal mechanics or from the additional stresses and strains created by the curve. So some degree of arthritis in the scoliotic spine is normal. The amount of arthritis associated with scoliosis does not, however, serve as an accurate predictor of the degree of pain a person will have.

What are the indications for treatment of scoliosis?

In general, orthopedists treat curves in growing youngsters that measure 25 to 30 degrees or more. The cutoff for size depends on the skeletal maturity of the patient: Older teenagers warrant treatment only if they have larger curves. Among adults, for whom the only effective treatment is surgery, the two indications for treatment are documented progression and/or pain consistent with the curve that proves unresponsive to nonoperative measures.

What types of treatment are available for scoliosis?

Observation, bracing, and surgery are the only methods used by orthopedists to treat scoliosis. Although other modalities may effectively relieve pain associated with scoliosis, they do not treat the scoliosis per se.

While a person is under observation for evidence of progression, should there be any restrictions on activity?

No. I encourage both children and adults to remain fully active without restrictions. In fact, I urge adults and children who are not physically active to increase their physical activity level, especially including those exercises that promote aerobic fitness. Adults with scoliosis may occasionally need to restrict their activity because of pain, but not for any other reason.

If I am under observation, how often do I need to see my orthopedist?

It depends on the age of the patient and the size of the curve. A 12-year-old with a 20-degree curve who has not yet begun to menstruate and is going through a rapid growth spurt should probably see her orthopedist every four months. A 15-year-old with a 20-degree curve who had her first menstrual cycle a year earlier may not need to see the orthopedist for a year. A 25-year-old with a 25-degree curve may require no follow-up at all unless she develops a problem later in life, because among adults, only curves in excess of 30 degrees have a significant risk of progression.

If one of my children has scoliosis, should I have my other children checked as well?

Yes. Siblings should be evaluated by either their pediatrician or an orthopedist. Typically, if I will be seeing a child with scoliosis for a follow-up visit, I ask the parents to bring their other children as well. This allows me to make a quick assessment without charging them anything extra for it.

If I have scoliosis, will my kids get it, too?

Since idiopathic scoliosis runs in families, your children will have an increased risk of developing it. But the genetic link is not simple, like hair color or eye color, making accurate predictions impossible. As a parent, you need to keep a close eye on your child's spine, watching carefully for any signs of development of the disease.

What can I do to minimize the risks associated with so many X-rays?

Radiologists now employ three techniques to reduce X-ray exposure. First, they focus the X-ray film entirely on the spine, so that the radiation exposure does not spread out to the rest of the body. Secondly, radiologists today use special "rare-earth" screens, a type of X-ray film that allows for a faster, shorter duration of exposure to X-rays. Finally, radiologists provide proper shielding: lead shields that minimize or entirely prevent exposure of the breasts, the thyroid, and the gonads.

In addition to these safeguards, you and your doctor can reduce your exposure by having X-rays taken only when absolutely necessary. Orthopedists initially use a scoliometer to determine the presence and estimate the magnitude of scoliosis, and only order X-rays if the scoliometer reading exceeds 6 degrees.

Lateral X-rays, those taken from the side, should be avoided unless the patient has a deformity in the normal front-to-back curve of the spine or will soon undergo surgery. Lateral X-rays require much more exposure because it takes more radiation to penetrate from side to side than it does from front to back. They also make it more difficult to shield those areas vulnerable to X-ray exposure. But most people with scoliosis don't need lateral X-rays on a routine basis.

What is the source of pain associated with scoliosis?

Scoliosis can cause a number of different kinds of pain. Mechanical, muscular pain results from decompensation — when the head doesn't line up over the center of the pelvis — caused by scoliotic curves. The muscles around the spine constantly make an effort to pull the individual back into compensation, which can lead to muscle fatigue and soreness. Pain might also arise due to compression of the facet joints in the concavity of the curve—i.e., the application of direct pressure on the facet joints. Radicular pain, pressure that results from a pinched nerve, typically in the concavity of the curve, is not uncommon among people who have scoliosis. In larger curves, the ribs may group together and press one on top of the other, which can also cause discomfort. Finally, pain may occur in the smaller curve below the major curve, typically as a result of arthritic degeneration.

Are there any surefire ways to treat chronic pain associated with scoliosis?

Although no one treatment will effectively reduce or manage pain for every patient, your doctor will try a number of different things to ease your pain. Exercise aimed at increasing strength and flexibility, back supports, and/or non-narcotic medication may help reduce the frequency, amount, and duration of your pain. (Narcotic medication should not be used to treat *chronic* pain, because it introduces the possibility of drug dependency.) A physical therapist might employ heat, ice, electrical stimulation, stretching, and/or other therapies to relieve pain. Chiropractic manipulation may also help alleviate an acute backache. You may also need to try lifestyle alterations: reducing physical activity or changing jobs, if necessary. All of these may help ease an acute backache. Unfortunately, for long-term chronic pain, these techniques may serve as little more than palliative measures: lessening the intensity of the pain, making it more bearable, but not eliminating it.

What is the value of exercise in treating scoliosis?

Exercise, though always beneficial, has absolutely *no* effect on the natural history of the disease. It will neither accelerate nor retard the progression of scoliosis. I encourage exercise on a regular basis to maintain physical and aerobic fitness. I may even prescribe a specific program of exercise for patients who have back pain. But these exercises promote general fitness and pain reduction, not curve reduction or the cessation of progression.

Is chiropractic effective in treating scoliosis?

Chiropractic manipulation will not affect the size of a scoliotic curve or the risk of progression. For people, particularly adults, who have sudden and acute back pain, chiropractic manipulation can sometimes help alleviate the pain. But chiropractors cannot reduce the size of a scoliotic curve. A chiropractor may improve the physical appearance of a scoliosis patient by, for example, giving a person a leg lift. Making the leg lengths unequal can compensate for the scoliotic curve's effect on the hips and thereby restore some symmetry. But clearly, adding further asymmetry to compensate for existing asymmetry does not really take care of the problem. It does nothing to reduce the curve or halt its progression.

Does electrical stimulation really work?

Many patients still ask about electrical stimulation, but this technique has been pretty much discredited. Double-blind randomized studies have shown that electrical stimulation doesn't appear to affect the natural history of the disease. The same percentage of cases get worse when treated with electrical stimulation as would get worse without any treatment whatsoever. This means electrical stimulation works as effectively as no treatment at all. The only difference is that electrical stimulation can cause complications such as skin irritations and sleep disturbances. So why use it?

What are the indications for bracing?

In general, the only people who wear a brace are those who have at least 18 months of growth remaining. In this case, curve size becomes the most important indication for bracing. Adolescents who achieve the best results from bracing are those with curves measuring between 30 and 39 degrees. Children with even smaller curves (25 degrees or more) should be considered suitable candidates for bracing where documented curve progression of 5 or more degrees exists. Young, skeletally immature children (Risser 0 or 1) might also be candidates for bracing at this magnitude. Bracing children with curves between 40 and 50 degrees has a 50 percent failure rate — but also a 50 percent success rate! So it remains an option, although a significantly less attractive one, with curves of this magnitude.

What is the goal of bracing?

The aim of bracing is to stop the progression of a curve, to keep a small curve small. Since their spines are flexible, kids tend to look straighter in the brace, but it will usually not afford any degree of permanent correction. Typically, once a patient has reached skeletal maturity and discontinued the brace, the spine will tend to sag back to where it started over the course of the next year or so.

What types of braces are available?

Although dozens of different braces exist, all fall into three basic categories. A variety of low-profile braces affix pressure pads to the inside of a plastic jacket that extends from under the arms down to the hips. The bulky Milwaukee brace consists of pressure pads held in place by vertical metal bars secured above by a neck ring and below by a pelvic girdle. The nighttime bending brace, which holds patients in a side-bending position, is not an ambulatory brace and should be worn only at night when the wearer is in a supine position.

How long will I need to wear a brace?

This depends on how young you are when you start wearing it and how effectively it works. If subsequent X-rays show that the brace has successfully halted progression of the curve, you will continue wearing the brace until you reach skeletal maturity. So a child put in a brace at age 8 might wear it for seven or eight years, while a child braced at age 13 might need it only for two or three years.

How many hours a day do I need to wear the brace?

This varies, depending on the size of the curve, the age of the patient, and the philosophy of the doctor. Some doctors simply don't believe in part-time bracing and will not use it under any circumstances. With full-time bracing, you will need to wear the brace 22 or 23 hours a day, taking the brace off only to shower and participate in gym class. I am convinced that part-time bracing does work well in many cases. Depending upon your age and curve size, a part-time bracing program might call on you to wear the brace 16 hours a day (meaning you don't have to wear it to school) or as little as 12 hours a day (in the evening and while you sleep). The Charleston nighttime bending brace is worn only 8 or 9 hours a day, while you sleep.

How successful is the nighttime bending brace compared to the others?

Since patients only wear it at night, they generally find the nighttime bending brace more tolerable than other braces and tend to comply more strictly to the bracing schedule. Most adolescents would therefore prefer a nighttime brace if they have to wear one. So how well does it work? Although limited preliminary studies suggest that they might work effectively, my own experience with nighttime bending braces has been disappointing. Though I have not prescribed it much, I have already seen it fail to halt progression several times. So I doubt its effectiveness, though conclusive evidence one way or the other has not yet been compiled.

Should any activities be restricted while I am in the brace?

You can do anything you want while wearing a brace, without restrictions of any kind. If you want to participate in specific after-school activities that bracing makes cumbersome—for example, dance or gymnastics—ask your doctor whether you can take the brace off for that additional hour or two. I would let you do so if you were my patient, even if you were on a full-time bracing program, but I am probably a little more lenient regarding bracing schedules than many other orthopedists. I don't think that an extra hour or two will have any significant impact on whether the brace will successfully halt progression, but it may make the brace a lot more tolerable psychologically.

If I undergo brace therapy, how long will I have to continue seeing the orthopedist?

If bracing treatment proves effective, I see children regularly, every four to six months, until they're skeletally mature. After discontinuing the brace, I usually have the patient return a year later for a follow-up examination and X-ray. If that X-ray looks good, I ask the patient to come back only every five years or so—unless a problem develops or the patient becomes pregnant. In either of these cases, the patient should consult an orthopedist and obtain a new X-ray (in the latter case, only *after* the pregnancy has been completed).

What are the indications for surgery?

Although indications differ somewhat depending upon the maturity of the patient, in general, the primary conditions that warrant surgery are a curve that exceeds 50 degrees, a rapidly progressing curve that exceeds 40 degrees and proved unresponsive to brace treatment, and/or severe and chronic pain associated with scoliosis.

Does scoliosis surgery need to be done right away?

Scoliosis surgery is never an emergency and can therefore always wait. Only documented rapid progression of a curve might indicate the need to do surgery relatively soon, say, within a couple of months. A 12-year-old whose curve has grown from 30 to 60 degrees in just six months should probably not wait too long to schedule surgery because the larger the curve grows, the less correction the surgeon can hope to achieve. On the other hand, a 25-year-old whose curve has progressed from 55 to 60 degrees over the last five years can wait five years or more before scheduling surgery.

It will ultimately make little difference whether the surgery is performed on a 60-degree curve or a 65-degree curve.

What are the alternatives to surgery?

In many cases, no reasonable alternatives exist if surgery is indicated. Among children, a small gray zone does exist for curve sizes in the high 30s or low 40s. Although the success rate for bracing may not be very high for such patients, it's still not an unreasonable alternative. All others who meet the indications for surgery, however, have only one choice: Either they have an operation or they don't.

What will spinal-fusion surgery do for me?

Spinal fusion stabilizes the back to obtain a correction and prevent progression further on in life. To accomplish this goal, the surgeon will need to stiffen a portion of the spine, in essence making it a solid bone rather than a flexible succession of independent vertebrae. Once the affected portion of the spine becomes solid bone, the curve should not progress any further.

Will I lose mobility as a result of spinal-fusion surgery?

Yes. Fusion stiffens part of the spine, eliminating motion between the targeted vertebral segments and creating the equivalent of a thigh bone in the back. For this reason, your surgeon will try to keep the fusion as short as possible, in some cases by suggesting an anterior rather than a posterior procedure. Although everyone who has a spinal fusion loses some motion, most people lose very little *functionally*. Those most likely to notice a functional difference include gymnasts, dancers, or others engaged in pursuits that demand excessive motion; those whose curves necessitate a very long fusion (i.e., 10 or more vertebrae); and those whose fusions extend to the lower lumbar spine.

What are the risks entailed by scoliosis surgery?

Surgery for scoliosis is in most cases safe, reliable, and predictable. But like any operation, it carries with it certain potential risks and complications: adverse reactions to anesthesia or pain medications, pneumonia and other medical complications, etc. Because the spine has a certain mystique about it, people worry more about spine surgery than about, say, leg surgery. Spine surgery requires bigger incisions and generally involves greater blood loss. But the thing that sets spine surgery apart more than anything else is the potential for damage to the spinal cord, which could lead to paralysis. Fortunately, the risk of paralysis or other serious spinal-cord injury is one in many, many thousands of operations. Especially in routine surgical cases for idiopathic scoliosis, the neurological risk is really very, very small.

Could I become paralyzed—or die—from this operation?

I have never had a patient paralyzed from surgery. As indicated above, the risk of paralysis from routine idiopathic scoliosis surgery is one in many thousands of cases.

Since most scoliosis patients are otherwise very healthy, typical postoperative complications will very, very rarely be fatal. The few complications that can be potentially lethal— for example, a pulmonary embolism—could result from any surgery, not just scoliosis surgery. Yet like paralysis, the risk of death from scoliosis surgery is one in many, many thousands of cases.

I don't think the risk of death or the risk of paralysis

should stop anyone from having this surgery, because both risks are so small. Although still very low, these risks do increase with more complicated types of scoliosis (neuromuscular or degenerative) or among older patients who already have medical problems. But even among these patients, the risk is very small—not zero perhaps, but very, very low.

How much will surgery correct my curve?

The average correction from posterior surgery is 50 to 60 percent. Larger, stiffer curves in adults afford less correction, perhaps around 40 percent. Operations on more flexible curves in younger people might achieve a 70 or 80 percent correction. Anterior procedures typically result in curve correction close to 80 percent.

What is overcorrection?

When a surgeon makes a scoliotic curve too straight, it can unbalance the patient. How can a correction be too straight? To avoid sacrificing too much mobility, surgeons fuse as few segments of the spine as possible, treating only the major structural curve. Yet most people with scoliosis also have smaller curves that have formed above and below the major curve. If these compensatory curves don't have enough inherent flexibility to compensate for the correction of the major curve, the latter has been overcorrected, and an imbalance results. Very small compensatory curves entail no risk of overcorrection: These patients will not become unbalanced. Overcorrecting a curve also increases the potential risk of spinal-cord damage. The more stress a surgeon puts on the spine to straighten it, the greater the potential for damage to the spinal cord. For this reason, surgeons aim for only a 40 percent correction in stiff, rigid curves, even though they routinely achieve a 70 or 80 percent correction in more flexible curves.

How long will the surgery take?

A typical posterior or anterior operation for scoliosis takes about three to four hours, plus another two hours or so for preparation, positioning, and recovery. Surgery on larger curves, longer curves, and older patients takes a little longer, as much as six or seven hours. Surgery that combines anterior and posterior procedures typically takes eight to ten hours. If the surgeon suspects it will take much longer than that, she will probably separate the procedures and perform two operations a week or two apart.

How serious is this operation?

Scoliosis surgery is a serious operation, a big operation, an invasive operation. But it is also a safe and reliable operation.

Why is instrumentation required?

Instrumentation—the rods as well as the hooks, clamps, wires, or screws that are attached directly to the spine—is needed to support the spine and hold it in position until the graft takes effect and the bones fuse. Instrumentation also often serves as the tool with which the surgeon achieves the correction. Without a solid bone fusion, however, the instrumentation will prove worthless.

I had Harrington-rod surgery in the 1970s: Is it really so outdated?

Though this method of treatment is no longer much used, I wouldn't worry unless you develop a problem. The vast majority of people with Harrington rods are doing just fine. Thousands and thousands of patients have received Harrington-rod instrumentation. Only a relatively small percentage have developed problems. Although the new systems are better, Harrington rods are a good tool, certainly the best that was available for many, many years. They're just not the best today.

Does the body ever reject instrumentation?

No. Rods are made of stainless steel or titanium and elicit no rejection response from the body. Rods and hardware can loosen, break, or become dislodged, necessitating removal. But in such cases, the body has not rejected them; they no longer fulfill their mechanical function.

Do hooks ever slip off the spine?

This can happen, although it occurred much more commonly with Harrington rods because this instrumentation used only two hooks. Today's multiple-hook and -screw devices, which employ many more points of fixation, put less stress on each hook, making them less likely to slip. I can't recall having had a single hook slip in ten years. If a hook does slip off the spine, it poses very little danger, but it might become more prominent and cause pain. Also, if the spine has not yet fused, the loss of fixation can lead to a loss of correction. This would necessitate repeating the procedure with more solid fixation.

Does the hardware have to come out sometime after the surgeon puts it in?

In general, no. Your surgeon will take the hardware out and, if necessary, reinstrument the spine only if the hardware is not doing what it's supposed to be doing because it breaks or becomes dislodged from the spine *and* the deformity recurs; or if the malfunctioning hardware causes pain or muscle irritation. If hardware breaks or dislodges after the spine has fused and it causes no pain, then it does not need to be taken out. In general, hardware is put in and left to stay.

What are pedicle screws and why are they so controversial?

Pedicle screws provide an alternative to hooks, clamps, and wires for anchoring instrumentation to the spine. Although not approved by the FDA, pedicle screws are a valuable tool, especially useful in fixing instrumentation to the spines of older patients whose poor bone quality makes the likelihood of fusion supported by any other type of fixation extremely unlikely. In the right hands, pedicle screws are safe and reliable, and in certain situations, they provide significant advantages.

What will a laminectomy do for me?

Your doctor will probably recommend a laminectomy if you have chronic and severe leg or back pain associated with scoliosis caused by spinal stenosis, which is the pinching of nerve roots caused by a narrowing of the spinal canal. This operation involves taking the roof off of the spinal canal to create adequate space for the nerves. A laminectomy is very rarely needed with idiopathic scolioses. Even among patients who do have some narrowing of the spinal canal, curve correction and the reduction of the deformity generally result in sufficient decompression of the canal. Laminectomy is more commonly indicated in degenerative scoliosis cases.

How long will I need to be in the hospital?

For either a posterior or an anterior procedure alone most people spend from five to eight days in the hospital. Combined procedures require a longer stay, closer to ten days.

What does the surgery feel like?

Having never experienced the surgery myself, I can't answer this question. I do know that it hurts, and that more extensive operations cause more pain. But pain is a very subjective sensation. The same operation can incapacitate one person with pain, while another person is up and about and smiling in a couple of days.

Is the surgery painful?

Again, it's a big operation and therefore always entails pain after surgery. Your doctor and the hospital staff will work very hard to control the pain with appropriate medication, but you will nonetheless feel some pain. But the pain always goes away in time. Incisional pain will begin to subside in a relatively short period of time. Graft pain can be a little more persistent, but in better than 95 percent of cases, will subside and not present a long-term problem.

What measures will be taken to manage this pain in the postoperative period?

Standard postoperative care employs a patient-controlled analgesic, a morphine pump that patients control themselves. A computer-driven, computer-controlled pump, the PCA delivers a certain predetermined amount of morphine at a steady rate. By pushing a button, you can give yourself additional morphine as needed up to a certain maximum, a limit set to prevent overdose. Typically, a PCA is used only for the first three or four days, when postoperative pain tends to be most severe. After that, you will take pain medications orally.

How long will I need to stay on painkillers?

Although you will probably need to continue taking narcotic pain medication for some time after surgery, you should be off all narcotics within a month or two. It would be inappropriate to continue narcotic pain medications any longer because of the danger of addiction, and I don't renew my patients' prescriptions at that point. Most adult patients stop on their own within about a month, while children almost never stay on narcotics for more than a week or two.

Will I look different after surgery?

Yes. All patients look different to a greater or lesser degree. The question you need to ask yourself is how important is this cosmetic result to you? Patients are commonly reluctant to talk about this, perhaps because they've been told that that's not what's important. But I think it *is* important. And it's important that you let your doctor know if it matters to you.

How will my physical appearance change?

You will be taller and your back will be straighter. But the other particulars of change depend on the specifics of your scoliosis. If you have a significant lumbar curve, your biggest cosmetic complaint probably concerns waistline asymmetry: One hip looks higher than the other. An anterior procedure will balance the hips and make the waist look virtually symmetrical. If you have a thoracic curve and your major cosmetic complaint centers around your rib hump, typical posterior surgery will provide only limited correction of the hump, about 15 to 17 percent. A thoracoplasty provides much better cosmetic results, correcting the rib hump by 70 or 80 percent. You need to let your doctor know how much your physical appearance matters to you, so he can choose the type of operation that best fulfills your needs.

Will I feel different after surgery?

Most patients who undergo scoliosis surgery ultimately view it as a very positive event in their lives. So I think most people do feel different. They feel better about themselves and more confident. They feel happy to have gone through this difficult experience and achieved a successful outcome.

Will I need a postoperative brace?

Probably not. I almost never prescribe postoperative braces. If a patient has weak bone, a determination that I make at the time of surgery, I might put that patient in a brace for three or four months. I also tend to use braces more often after revision surgery because it protects the hardware, making it a little more secure. But even with revision surgeries, braces are not generally needed.

How active will I be immediately after surgery?

On the day after surgery, you will not be at all active. Although I would encourage you to do whatever you feel like doing, you won't feel like doing much. Your activity will gradually increase during your stay in the hospital: sitting up on the second day; standing on the second or third day; walking on the third or fourth day; and, generally, walking gingerly but without assistance by discharge.

When can I shower after surgery?

Typically, postsurgical patients can start showering without worrying about getting the incision wet after about five days.

What will I be able to do when I go home?

By the time you are discharged from the hospital, you will be able to walk short distances, go up and down some stairs, go out of the house, ride in a car, and do anything else you feel comfortable doing. You will probably not feel up to cleaning the house, washing the car, shopping, or mowing the lawn. For a couple of months, you will need help with more strenuous activities such as these.

When can I resume sexual relations?

Whenever you feel comfortable doing so, you can resume sexual activity. However, you may need to adjust or modify the way you enjoy sex because certain positions or activities may be painful for a while.

When will I be able to drive again?

Most patients can start to drive again within a few weeks or a month, whenever they feel comfortable. However, you should initially limit your driving to short distances—less than half an hour at a time.

How long will I be out of school?

If you have your operation during the school term, you can probably return to school after a month or six weeks. Some kids go back after just three weeks, or even two. If you have your operation early in the summer, you will be back in school on schedule in the fall.

Will I be able to participate fully in school activities?

Yes, but not right away. I often keep patients out of gym for a semester and discourage after-school sports during this period as well.

When can I return to work?

This obviously depends on what kind of work you do and what kind of surgical procedure was performed. Adults who have fairly sedentary work and have undergone a straightforward anterior or posterior surgery require a minimum of six weeks before returning to work and more commonly need three to six months. Those who have had both front and back surgery commonly need six to twelve months. Some of my patients have gotten back to work sooner than that, but if you're asking for a time frame that you can plan your life around, it's better to err on the side of caution.

When can I pick up my baby again?

Again, it depends upon the surgical procedure and is more a matter of comfort than danger. When you first go home, you will not be able to handle every aspect of child care. Certainly you can hold and cuddle your baby, you can take care of the child in many respects, but picking up the baby or toddler, especially lifting her out of the crib, will just be too uncomfortable for the first month or two. So if you have small children, you will need some extra help during this time.

Having scoliosis, will I be able to have children?

Absolutely. In most cases, scoliosis has no effect whatsoever on the ability to conceive or carry a pregnancy to term. Only women with curves so severe that they have caused significant cardiorespiratory problems should consider avoiding pregnancy because it might overtax the already damaged heart and lungs. But curves that exceed 100 degrees, the size that would cause cardiorespiratory problems, are almost never seen today. Spinal fusion, although it does not affect the ability to conceive or carry a pregnancy, has been associated with a slightly increased incidence of Caesarean sections. This increase is minimal, however, and may result as much from the way the obstetrician manages these patients as from the fusion itself. Perhaps obstetricians consider them less able to undergo the back strain of vaginal delivery.

Since pregnancy can put a strain on the back, I generally advise postoperative scoliosis patients to wait six months before trying to get pregnant. I've had patients who have become pregnant before that and to my knowledge none has had any problem with her pregnancy. But I would prefer patients wait six months in order to give the spine a chance to fuse without the extra load of pregnancy.

How long will I need to continue seeing the orthopedist after my surgery?

After discharge from the hospital, I generally see my patients four to six weeks after surgery to check the fusion and see if any problems have arisen. I next see them at three months, at which time I let them be fully active except for contact sports or activities that risk a bad fall. The third post-op visit is at six months, at which point I tell patients that they can be fully active without restriction. I also see patients a year after surgery, to make sure they have fused properly. I then ask them to come back annually for the next four years. At each postoperative visit I order X-rays, typically an A-P and a lateral. After the last visit, five years post-op, my patients need to come back only if there's a problem.

What's the long-term prognosis, 30 or 40 years down the road, for people who have scoliosis surgery?

People who have had scoliosis, whether or not it was severe enough to warrant surgery, will never have normal backs. Even after successful surgery you may still have more deformity, more pain, and/or less work and recreational tolerance than someone who never had scoliosis or never required surgery for it. However, if you had appropriate and successful surgery, you will almost certainly have less deformity, less pain, and higher work and recreational tolerance than you would have without the surgery.

How active can I be when I'm fully healed?

You can do whatever you're comfortable doing. Once the spine has fused, I don't restrict a patient's activity at all. Children and adults can play any sports they want to. You will have no work restrictions in terms of lifting or carrying. You may find that you can't do everything you'd like, but I wouldn't restrict you from anything you want to do.

What are the kids who have had this surgery like?

Most kids view themselves as perfectly normal. They do everything they want to do without restrictions of any kind.

Will I be able to have a normal life—play sports and have children and do all those physical things?

Yes. That's the expected result of surgery: You can do anything.

Scoliosis Organizations and Associations

American Academy of Orthopaedic Surgeons
6300 N. River Road
Rosemont, IL 60018-4262
(800) 346-2267
Fax (708) 823-8026

National Scoliosis Foundation, Inc.
72 Mount Auburn Street
Watertown, MA 02172
(617) 926-0397
Fax: (617) 926-0398
E-mail: Scoliosis@aol.com

The Scoliosis Association, Inc.
P.O. Box 811705
Boca Raton, FL 33481-1705
(800) 800-0669
Fax: (407) 368-8518

Scoliosis Research Society
6300 N. River Road
Suite 727
Rosemont, IL 60018-4226
(708) 698-1627
Fax: (708) 823-0536

APPENDIX B

Recommended Reading

Although we know of only one other nonfiction book on scoliosis suitable for nonprofessional audiences, a number of pamphlets, most of them published by the organizations listed in Appendix A, are available to patients and their families, children and adults alike:

Adult Spinal Deformity: Scoliosis and Kyphosis, A Patient's Handbook. Park Ridge, Ill.: Scoliosis Research Society, 1987.

Coonrad, Ralph W. *Which Twin Has Scoliosis?* Raleigh, N.C.: North Carolina Department of Human Resources, Division of Health Services, Developmental Disabilities Branch, 1987.

Fenner, Louise. *When the Spine Curves*. Rockville, Md.: Department of Health and Human Services, Public Health Service, Food and Drug Administration, 1985. (HE 20.4010/a-Sp 4).

Questions Most Often Asked of the National Scoliosis Foundation, Inc. Belmont, Mass.: National Scoliosis Foundation, Inc., 1995.

Schommer, Nancy. *Stopping Scoliosis: The Complete Guide to Diagnosis and Treatment*. New York: Doubleday, 1987.

Scoliosis: A Handbook for Patients. Park Ridge, Ill.: Scoliosis Research Society, 1986.

Scoliosis and Kyphosis: Information and Advice for Parents. Park Ridge, Ill.: Scoliosis Research Society, 1986.

Glossary

A-P X-Rays Anteroposterior X-rays, taken with the patient facing the X-ray machine, increasing the exposure of breast tissue to radiation, but decreasing the exposure of the pelvis and bone marrow.

apical translation A surgical technique of curve correction that involves moving the apex of a scoliotic curve closer to the midline of the back.

arthritis Inflammation and enlargement of the joints, often marked by the formation of bone spurs as the body tries to heal the inflammation.

cervical vertebrae The seven vertebrae of the neck; the cervical vertebrae connect the thoracic, or chest, portion of the spine to the skull.

Cobb angle The standard measure for scoliotic curves; derived by drawing lines parallel to the top and bottom vertebrae of a curve, drawing lines perpendicular to these two original lines, and measuring the angle of intersection of these perpendiculars.

coccyx The lowest segment of the spinal column; also called the tailbone.

compensation Overall balance throughout the length of the spine, so that the head is centered over the pelvis. Compensation is the primary goal of scoliosis surgery.

computerized axial tomography A diagnostic tool, more commonly known as a CAT scan, that employs X-ray sweeps to produce clear, detailed cross-sectional images of internal structures such as the spine.

congenital scoliosis Scoliosis present at birth as a result of abnormalities in the spinal column that cause it to grow asymmetrically.

decompensation   Any degree of imbalance in the spine that results in the head not being centered over the pelvis.

degenerative scoliosis   Scoliosis that develops in a previously straight spine during adulthood owing to degeneration of discs *(q.v.)*, arthritis in the facet joints *(q.v.)*, and/or loss of support in the spinal column.

disc   A fibrous cartilage ring that surrounds a soft, spongy core (the nucleus pulposus) and rests between two vertebrae; the discs function as shock absorbers for the spine.

distraction   A surgical technique of curve correction that involves pulling the ends of a curve farther apart.

facet joints   Joints located at the back of the spine that unite the vertebrae. Each vertebra has two facet joints: The inferior one joins with the vertebra below; the superior one joins with the vertebra above.

fusion   A surgical technique, used to maintain correction and halt progression of a scoliotic curve, that involves fusing independent vertebrae into a solid mass of bone.

graft   In scoliosis surgery, bone chips, usually taken from the ilium or a rib, used to promote the healing and fusion of bone.

idiopathic scoliosis   Scoliosis of unknown origin. The most common type of scoliosis, it can first appear in early childhood or adulthood, but most commonly presents itself initially during adolescence.

ileus   An obstruction of the bowel that causes distension and pain in the abdomen and is a common complication of scoliosis surgery.

ilium   The hindmost pelvic bone.

instrumentation   Hardware used to achieve internal fixation of scoliotic curve correction.

internal fixation   A surgical technique that employs foreign supports, generally metal rods, to correct and stabilize the spine while the bone heals and fuses.

kyphosis   The normal rounding of the upper part of the back when viewed from the side. Kyphosis is sometimes flattened as a result of scoliosis or of treatment for scoliosis.

lateral   From side to side, the primary deviation of scoliotic curves.

lordoscoliosis   A flattening of the thoracic kyphosis that sometimes accompanies scoliosis.

lordosis The normal concavity of the lower part of the back when viewed from the side. Lordosis is sometimes flattened as a result of scoliosis or of treatment for scoliosis.

lumbar decompression A surgical technique, also called *lumbar laminectomy*, used to correct spinal stenosis by taking off the lamina (roof of the spinal canal) in order to provide more space for the nerves.

lumbar discography An unpleasant but sometimes necessary diagnostic test that can help determine the source of back pain caused by degenerative scoliosis by injecting fluid into each suspected disc and seeing which ones produce the pain congruent with the patient's symptomatic complaint.

lumbar vertebrae The seven vertebrae that make up the lower back, rising from the sacrum to the thoracic spine.

magnetic resonance imaging (MRI) A diagnostic tool that uses a powerful magnetic field to provide a clear, detailed, three-dimensional view of internal structures.

myelogram A diagnostic test used to trace neural pathways and discover the sources of spinal stenosis or other nerve problems by injecting dye into the spinal canal prior to taking X-rays and/or performing a CAT scan.

orthotist A manufacturer of orthotic devices such as the braces used to inhibit the progression of scoliosis.

osteoporosis A condition, marked by brittle or porous bones, due to the loss of calcium.

osteotomy Surgically fracturing—cutting through—bone in order to promote realignment and refusion in a better position.

P-A X-rays Posteroanterior (back-to-front) X-rays, taken with the patient facing away from the X-ray machine, allowing the body to shield breast tissue from most radiation, but increasing the exposure of the pelvis and bone marrow.

pedicle screw A device, not approved by the FDA, sometimes used to secure instrumentation to the spine.

progression An increase of 5 or more degrees in curve magnitude, as measured by X-ray.

pseudorarthrosis Failure of spinal fusion, resulting in continued mobility in an area that should no longer move.

revision surgery   Surgery performed on someone who has already had surgery.

sacrum   A section of naturally fused vertebrae that lies between the lumbar spine and the coccyx.

sagittal curves   Curves (kyphosis and lordosis) present in a normal spine seen when the spine is viewed from the side.

scoliometer   A simple tool for scoliosis screening that measures the degree of inclination of a rib hump and thereby detects rib rotation.

scoliosis   The presence of a lateral deviation of 10 degrees or more in the spine, often associated with rotation of the vertebrae.

spinal claudication   Disabling cramping in the legs, caused by nerve-root entrapment in the spine, which is the signature symptom of spinal stenosis.

spinal stenosis   A narrowing or constriction of the spinal canal that results in the entrapment of nerves; it is a secondary condition common among patients with degenerative scoliosis.

spondylolisthesis   The slippage and separation of one vertebra from the one under it, often due to degeneration and consequent incompetence of discs and facet joints. Spondylolisthesis can create a curve that resembles scoliosis.

spondylosis   Arthritis of the spine, a common complication of advanced scoliosis.

thoracic vertebrae   The 12 vertebrae that make up the middle and upper back and support the rib cage.

thoracoplasty   A surgical technique that involves cutting away part of one or more ribs involved in a significant rib hump.

vertebrae   Twenty-four flexible bony elements that, with the sacrum and coccyx, form the human spinal column.

wake-up test   A test used to detect any possible neurological damage during surgery by decreasing the level of anesthesia to the point where patients wake up, wiggle their toes, and are then put back to sleep. Although performed before closing the incision, patients do not feel pain and generally do not even remember the test.

Index